FOOD CHOICE AND OBESITY
IN BLACK AMERICA

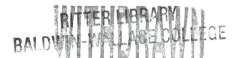

FOOD CHOICE AND OBESITY
IN BLACK AMERICA

Creating a New Cultural Diet

Eric J. Bailey

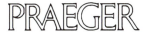

Westport, Connecticut
London

Library of Congress Cataloging-in-Publication Data

Bailey, Eric J., 1958
  Food choice and obesity in Black America : creating a new
cultural diet / Eric J. Bailey.
     p. cm.
  Includes bibliographical references and index.
  ISBN 0–86569–330–7 (alk. paper)

  1. Obesity—United States. 2. Food preferences—United States. 3. African
Americans—Health and hygiene—Social aspects. 4. Reducing diets—Social
aspects. I. Title.
  RC628.B282 2006
   362.196'39800896073—dc22   2006001234

British Library Cataloguing in Publication Data is available.

This book is included in the African American Experience database from
Greenwood Electronic Media. For more information, visit
www.africanamericanexperience.com.

Library of Congress Catalog Card Number: 2006001234
ISBN: 0–86569-330-7

First published in 2006

Praeger Publishers, 88 Post Road West, Westport, CT 06881
An imprint of Greenwood Publishing Group, Inc.
www.praeger.com

Printed in the United States of America

The paper used in this book complies with the
Permanent Paper Standard issued by the National
Information Standards Organization (Z39.48–1984).

10 9 8 7 6 5 4 3 2 1

This book is dedicated to my wife—Gloria Jean Harden Bailey. After the birth of our second child, Darrien, and the relocation from Atlanta, Georgia, back to a Midwestern city, Gloria noticed that I had put on some extra pounds and looked very bloated. In fact, I had to purchase a new set of larger pants because my waistline and stomach area had substantially increased during this period. I was amazed and in denial because I was still exercising and following my particular health regimen. Although all of us, including my daughter Ebony, laughed about my heavier weight, it became increasingly a concern for us, particularly when the excess weight caused my blood pressure to increase. After several different types of health, fitness, and diet regimens, and a move from Little Rock, Arkansas, to a Mid-Atlantic town in Maryland, I realized that I needed a health, fitness, and diet program that truly fits me—a 47-year-old, African American man. With Gloria's insight, expertise, experience, and encouragement, I began to formulate this new approach to diet, health, and physical fitness for not only myself but for all African Americans. Although our culture embraces a more flexible definition of what constitutes a "healthy" person, we as African Americans have been in denial about our overweight and obesity issues for decades, and I believe that we are experiencing needless overweight and obesity health consequences such as diabetes, hypertension, asthma, cancer, and death. Therefore, this book is dedicated to my wife—Gloria Jean Harden Bailey.

CONTENTS

Preface ix

Acknowledgments xi

Part I. The African American Overweight and Obesity Problem

1. The African American Weight Problem 3

2. Overweight and Obesity among African Americans 23

Part II. Sociocultural Issues

3. Body Image Preferences among African Americans 43

4. Food Preferences among African Americans 61

5. Exercise and Physical Fitness Perspectives
   among African Americans 81

6. Adding African American Culture to Health, Physical
   Fitness, Diet, and Food Programs 105

Part III. The New Cultural Approach

7. The New Black Cultural Diet and Lifestyle 131

Appendix: Useful Sources 153

Bibliography 157

Index 167

PREFACE

Food Choice and Obesity in Black America is a book that attempts to be the first in examining comprehensively and, particularly, culturally the overweight and obesity issues in the African American community; the first in taking a holistic and cultural historic approach to African Americans' food preferences, particularly soul food; the first in highlighting African Americans' preferences for body image, body type, and body build; the first in examining African Americans' perspective on physical fitness and exercise; and the first in providing a cultural framework for all other health and fitness and diet programs that strive to be successful in the African American community. Whether this book is actually the first in all these topics is not the issue, but what is the issue is that all of us need to look at overweight and obesity in all the African American communities—the higher socioeconomic community, the middle socioeconomic community, and the lower socioeconomic community—much more seriously, once and for all!

Chapter 1 is a wake-up call to African Americans about the issues of being overweight and obese. This chapter highlights a personal story of an African American family struggling with diabetes and weight loss; it also addresses the *cultural pattern* of "being bigger and fat is okay"; it highlights a state's public health strategy for addressing overweight and obesity in the African American community, and it highlights one of my research studies investigating the chronic effects of overweight and obesity in the African American population.

The facts and foundation regarding the medical and health consequences of being overweight and obese in our society are established in

Chapter 2. This chapter provides the scientific data and reports on life expectancy and major causes of mortality and morbidity in the United States; it highlights the current data on overweight and obesity in the U.S. population; it shows the current data on overweight and obesity among children in the U.S. population; and it concludes with stating the current data on overweight and obesity among African Americans.

How African Americans view their body image is examined in Chapter 3. This chapter highlights African Americans' preferences for ideal body type; it defines overweight, obesity, and body mass index from the public health perspective; it reviews several research studies on African Americans body type and body image preferences; and it suggests that African Americans have a *flexible cultural definition of healthiness.*

The strong relationship that African Americans have with their particular food preferences is recognized in Chapter 4. This chapter reviews several well-known *soul food* cookbooks; it examines the cultural history of African American cuisine; it defines *soul food;* it discusses food, food habits and present-day African American cuisine; and it highlights my personal and cultural connection with *soul food.*

Chapter 5 describes how African Americans feel about exercise and fitness programs. This chapter addresses corporate America's lack of health and fitness items for the African American market; it highlights several research studies on physical fitness and African Americans; and it highlights how I developed my exercise and fitness regimen.

Culture is introduced to diet and physical fitness programs in Chapter 6. This chapter defines culture; it discusses why culture is important to diet and physical fitness programs for African Americans; it defines African American culture; it reviews several research studies emphasizing the important role of African American culture in diet and physical fitness programs; it highlights successful federal diet and fitness programs that used African American culture; and it reviews other successful diet and physical fitness books that embraced African American culture.

Finally, Chapter 7 introduces the New Black Cultural Diet™. This chapter defines *cultural appropriateness;* it highlights specific culturally appropriate overweight and obesity intervention for specific segments of the African American population; it covers the major cultural health and fitness questions; and it provides my strategy for using the key components of the New Black Cultural Diet™.

Acknowledgments

It has been my pleasure and joy to complete my third book for Greenwood Publishing over the past six years. I want to sincerely thank my editor, Debora Carvalko, and all the staff at Greenwood Publishing.

Now that I have returned to academia, I want to thank two federal institutions for allowing me to become a part of their culture. They are the National Institutes of Health, where I served as a Health Scientist Administrator at the National Cancer Institute, and the National Center on Minority Health and Health Disparities. I also want to thank the Centers for Disease Control and Prevention, where I served as a Postdoctoral Fellow in HIV/AIDS in the Tuberculosis Division and the Office of Minority Health. Moreover, the National Library of Medicine at the National Institutes of Health has been an invaluable resource for all of my past, present, and future research endeavors.

In addition, I want to thank the various academic institutions that provided me opportunities for research, teaching, service, and leadership. They are Miami University (Ohio), Central State University (Ohio), Wayne State University (Michigan), Indiana University at Indianapolis (IUPUI), Emory University, University of Arkansas for Medical Sciences (UAMS), Charles R. Drew University of Medicine and Science, and, of course, East Carolina University (North Carolina).

Naturally, there are several key scholars and health administrators who I want to recognize for assisting me with my recent career and research ideals. They are Sandra Millon Underwood, Richard Levinson, Jean Flagg-Newton, Lorrita Watson, Vincent Thomas, Holly Matthews, Linda Wolfe, Rick Ward, and John Ruffin.

As always, I give my respect and guidance to my family members, past and present: my phenomenal mother, Jean Ethel Bailey; father, Roger Bailey; and brothers, Dwight, Ronnie, Billie, and Michael Bailey.

Finally, I want to thank my very supportive family for following me around from state to state—my wife, Gloria; daughter, Ebony; and sons, Darrien and Marcus.

PART I

THE AFRICAN AMERICAN OVERWEIGHT AND OBESITY PROBLEM

The first section of this book is a wake-up call to African Americans about the issues of being overweight and obese. The latest findings, reports, definitions, and scientific data on overweight and obesity are presented as they relate to the African American population.

THE AFRICAN AMERICAN WEIGHT PROBLEM

Critical Thinking Questions

1. Why do African Americans have a weight problem?
2. Does overweight contribute to other major health problems?
3. Why don't African Americans recognize the relationship of being overweight with other health problems like diabetes?
4. Is there a different view or perspective as to what constitutes "overweight" in the African American population?

Introduction

I want to begin this book with a personal account from an African American family that is fighting this problem of overweight and obesity. I became aware of this family's ordeal when their story was published in the weekend edition of *USA Weekend* (November 15–17, 2002). Their story was the fifth in a series of stories on families seeking medical and health advice from a physician (Dr. Tedd Mitchell).

The article, entitled "Keep Moving Toward the Lite," centers around an African American mother (Brenda Tutt, age 55) who recently was diagnosed with type 2 diabetes and who already suffers from hypertension and osteoarthritis. She is attempting to fight her overweight and obesity problem with the help of her family. Her husband (Godwin Tutt, age 57) has been diagnosed with mild hypertension, and he is attempting to quit

3

smoking. Finally, her daughter (Jennifer Tutt, age 21) is in good health and exercises regularly.

What is so fascinating about their story? It is quite similar to that of so many African American families across America, involving as it does a recently retired professional like Brenda Tutt, a recently retired husband like Godin Tutt, and a daughter who is going to college but feels a family commitment to help her mother lose the weight by staying home and commuting to college. Thus, the Tutt family is very typical of a lot of African American families who have worked hard for their companies, finally retire from their companies, have a child attending college, yet while in retirement are diagnosed with a weight-related medical problem such as type 2 diabetes.

As Dr. Tedd Mitchell (2002) describes Brenda's situation, the major issues are as follows:

- Brenda wants to avoid medication for diabetes, so she's controlling her blood sugar through portion control and diet.
- Brenda knows that to improve her health risks, she needs to lose weight.
- To lose weight she needs to exercise.
- But exercise causes knee pain.
- Less exercise means more weight gain.
- And more weight gain means worse health risks. (Mitchell 2002: 6)

Although the weight problem and diabetes status may appear to be too daunting to overcome, Dr. Tedd suggested that the Tutts should keep this motto in mind: *Simple things done consistently is the way to go.* Because Mrs. Tutt has a lot going for her—a vibrant family, a successful career, and fulfilling volunteer work—she has a better than average chance to succeed in making lifestyle changes that assist in losing weight and improving her quality of life.

To reiterate, this African American story is very typical of other African American stories across the United States. The fact that African Americans are developing more weight-related diseases such as type 2 diabetes, hypertension, and cancers suggests that we are not connecting the two issues (overweight and chronic disease), and also we are not addressing and developing long-term solutions for the issues of overweight and obesity in our communities (Satcher 2001).

The Facts About Diabetes Mellitus

What Is Diabetes?

Diabetes mellitus is a group of diseases characterized by high levels of blood glucose. It results from defects in insulin secretion, insulin action, or both. Diabetes mellitus occurs in four forms classified by etiology: type 1 (insulin-dependent), type 2 (non–insulin-dependent), other special types (genetic disorder or exposure to certain drugs in chemicals), and gestational diabetes (occurs during pregnancy). Diabetes can be associated with serious complications and premature death, but people with diabetes can take measures to reduce the likelihood of such occurrences.

Most African Americans (about 90% to 95%) with diabetes have type 2 diabetes. This type of diabetes usually develops in adults and is caused by the body's resistance to the action of insulin and to impaired insulin secretion. It can be treated with diet, exercise, diabetes pills, and injected insulin. A small number of African Americans (about 5% to 10%) have type 1 diabetes, which usually develops before age 20 and is always treated with insulin.

Diabetes can be diagnosed by three methods:

- A fasting plasma glucose test with a value of 126 milligrams/deciliter (mg/dL) or greater
- A nonfasting plasma glucose value of 200 mg/dL or greater in people with symptoms of diabetes
- An abnormal oral glucose tolerance test with a 2-hour glucose value of 200 mg/dL or greater

Each test must be confirmed, on another day, by any one of the above methods (National Institute of Diabetes and Digestive and Kidney Diseases [NIDDK] 2005).

Current Statistics and Health Impact in the African American Population

Today, diabetes mellitus is one of the most serious health challenges facing the African American population. According to the National Institute of Diabetes and Digestive and Kidney Disorders (NIDDK) at the National Institutes of Health (NIH), the following statistics illustrate the magnitude of this disease among African Americans.

- 2.8 million African Americans have diabetes
- On average, African Americans are twice as likely to have diabetes as white Americans of similar age

- Approximately 13 percent of all African Americans have diabetes

- African Americans with diabetes are more likely to develop diabetes complications and experience greater disability from the complications than white Americans with diabetes

- Death rates for people with diabetes are 27 percent higher for African Americans compared with whites

National health surveys during the past 35 years show that the percentage of the African American population that has been diagnosed with diabetes is increasing dramatically. In 1976–1980, total diabetes prevalence in African Americans ages 40 to 74 years was 8.9 percent; in 1988–1994, total prevalence had increased to 18.2 percent—a doubling of the rate in just 12 years.

Overall, among those age 20 years or older, the rate is 11.8 percent for women and 8.5 percent for men. About one-third of total diabetes cases are undiagnosed among African Americans. This is similar to the proportion for other racial/ethnic groups in the United States.

Compared with white Americans, African Americans experience higher rates of diabetes complications such as eye disease, kidney failure, and amputations. They also experience greater disability from these complications. Some factors that influence the frequency of these complications, such as high blood glucose levels, abnormal blood lipids, high blood pressure, and cigarette smoking, can be influenced by proper diabetes management.

The frequency of diabetes in African American adults is influenced by the same risk factors that are associated with type 2 diabetes in other populations. Two categories of risk factors increase the chance of developing type 2 diabetes. The first is genetics. The second is medical and lifestyle risk factors, including impaired glucose tolerance, gestational diabetes, hyperinsulinemia and insulin resistance, physical inactivity, and obesity.

Overweight is a major risk factor for type 2 diabetes. In addition to the overall level of obesity, the location of the excess weight is also a risk factor for type 2 diabetes. Excess weight carried above the waist is a stronger risk factor than excess weight carried below the waist. African Americans have a greater tendency to develop upper-body obesity, which increases their risk of diabetes (National Institute of Diabetes and Digestive and Kidney Diseases [NIDDK] 2005).

My Research Study Related to Diet and Health: The Diabetes Study and African Americans

Background Information

As a population, African Americans are at increased risk for developing diabetes mellitus. African Americans also experience higher rates of at least three of the serious complications of diabetes: blindness, amputations, and end-stage renal disease. The primary objective of this study was to assess the relationship between health beliefs and patterns of health service utilization in two populations with non–insulin-dependent diabetes that are economically similar but culturally different: African Americans and European Americans. In cooperation with the Regenstrief Health Center at Indiana University, the research team conducted a two-year qualitative and quantitative study to examine the health beliefs and health care seeking pattern of African American and European American diabetic patients. Qualitative findings were as follows: (1) assess the patient's cause of the diabetes; (2) attempt to address any misconception of diabetes; and (3) adjust the diabetic regimen to the individual's social and ethnic lifestyle pattern (Bailey 2002).

In 1991, I was contacted by the Indiana University Diabetes Research and Training Center to assist a team of researchers who wanted to investigate the role that culturally influenced health beliefs play in both disease status and health service utilization of African Americans with non–insulin-dependent diabetes (NIDDM) or type 2 diabetes mellitus. Once I met with the project director (physician) and the team of behavioral scientists in the School of Medicine, I felt that I could contribute substantially to the intervention phase of this study.

My specific goals were (1) to develop and to validate a health belief assessment tool that is responsive to the cultural perspectives of African Americans and (2) to administer the health belief assessment tool to two NIDDM patient samples and determine the relationship between the patients' beliefs and actual usage of health care services. It was expected that the health belief assessment tool would be incorporated into the data collection for the larger-scale study under way and that the instrument could assist in predicting adherence to the diabetes regimens in this population.

In order to accomplish the specific goals, I designed a three-phase approach to my study: (1) conduct a five-month qualitative study of patients attending the Diabetes Clinic (June 1, 1991 to October 31, 1991); (2) conduct a three-month qualitative and quantitative study of African American and European American patients attending the Diabetes Clinic (June 1, 1992 to August 31, 1992); and (3) test and analyze a quantitative and qualitative culturally sensitive assessment tool.

During phase 1, in cooperation with the Regenstrief Health Center and the Diabetes Research and Training Center, I conducted a five-month study of patients attending the Diabetes Clinic. Qualitative observations and informal interviews were gathered from physicians, nurses, staff members, and patients in an attempt not only to comprehensively understand the sociocultural dynamics of the diabetic patient but also to prepare the principal investigator for conducting a clinically applied anthropological study.

The diabetes patient population was selected from the diabetes population treated at the Wishard Memorial Hospital located on the Indiana University Medical School campus (Regenstrief Health Center). Wishard Memorial Hospital is a 540-bed general medical/surgical hospital that primarily serves the inner-city residents of Indianapolis. It is owned by the county Health and Hospital Corporation and is operated by the Indiana University School of Medicine.

Phase 2 consisted of qualitative observations, informal interviews, and semistructured interviews of patients in the Diabetes Clinic. The primary purpose of phase 2 was to determine patients' perceptions of the cause of the diabetic condition and symptoms and common side effects of their diabetic treatment regimen. Interviews were conducted with subjects in an outpatient clinic setting after they completed their scheduled clinic appointment.

The semistructured questionnaire was used to assess the health beliefs and health care seeking pattern of the diabetic patient. Items that significantly predicted variance were used in construction of the African American Health Belief Inventory (AAHBI©). The AAHIBI was based upon subjects' responses to the following instruments:

1.   Health Belief Model;
2.   Diabetes Symptom Questionnaire;
3.   Medical care satisfaction; and
4.   A structured clinical interview.

Phase 3 consisted of testing and determining the effectiveness of the African American Health Belief Inventory on two samples—African Americans and European Americans—with similar duration of non–insulin-dependent diabetes and similar age, sex, and socioeconomic standing. Quantitative data from the AAHBI were integrated with qualitative interviews to produce a holistic view of the sociodemographic, psychosocial, and cultural factors that influence the African American diabetic health care seeking pattern.

Research Findings

Stage 1: Qualitative Results

The first stage of my diabetes study consisted only of observations and informal interviews of patients, physicians, and staff members in the Diabetes Clinic, beginning June 11, 1991. Once I arrived at the clinic (8:30 a.m.), I immediately began my observations.

In addition to the observations of the clinic, I conducted informal interviews with patients, physicians, nurses, and staff members during the first day. The following points best describe the major qualitative issues of concern to patients, physicians, and nurses:

1. Because physicians rotate to different clinics, patients rarely see the same physician twice.

2. Patients are often referred to another specialist and another clinic.

3. Patient adherence to prescribed diabetic regimen is very low.

4. Patients often arrive with a family member or friend.

5. Patients' perceptions of their diabetes are often different from what the physician has told them.

6. Physicians expect degrees of difficulty for patients to adhere to diabetic regimen.

On this first day, for example, informal interviews with two patients highlighted their predicaments and strategies for adhering to the diabetic regimen. While sitting in the patient area, I started a conversation with a middle-aged African American female (patient informant no. 1). After I informed her of my study, she agreed to share her story with me. Her story is summarized as follows:

Patient Informant No. 1: Patient informant no. 1 discovered her diabetic condition by accident. It happened when she cut her foot accidentally. After several weeks passed, her foot did not heal properly. She sought care from her regular doctor, and he diagnosed her diabetes. She was later referred to this Diabetes Clinic. Although she knew that other family members had developed diabetes, she did not think that she was susceptible. Patient informant no. 1 also felt that she did not need any assistance in her daily activities but later had to admit that she needed help from family members. Because her son lives with her, her daughter lives next door, and she has close friends in the neighborhood, she has a high degree of support from her network of family members and friends. Her motto is to "live each day one day at a time."

By 12:27 p.m., I had completed my first day of observations and informal interviews at the Diabetes Clinic. This day was typical of all the remaining site visits that I conducted during the next five months.

From the nine total site visits over the five months, the following themes were significant with regard to the African American diabetic patient:

1. Assess the patient's cause of the diabetes.

2. Attempt to dispel any misconceptions of diabetes.

3. Activate the patient for self-care diabetes.

4. Continue to reeducate the patient on blood glucose monitoring and insulin injection.

5. Encourage social and familial support for adherence to diabetic regimen.

In addition, other qualitative results indicated that physicians need to:

1. Understand the sociocultural constraints of a patient's keeping of appointments;

2. Adjust the dietary modification of the patient to his or her lifestyle and ethnic dietary pattern;

3. Develop more continuity of care;

4. Learn new skills to develop rapport and trust with patients; and

5. Emphasize the seriousness of the diabetic condition to the patient.

Stage 2: Qualitative Results and Semistructured Interviews

Stage 2 consisted of conducting qualitative and quantitative observations and interviews of African American and Euro-American diabetic patients. For example, during the three-month portion of stage 2, African American patients shared the following comments:

> "Patient Informant No. 3 (African American male): I believe that my diabetes is due to the stress that I endure each and every day. My lifestyle is uncertain and unpredictable, so I think that the stress that I am under caused my diabetes."

Although patient informant no. 3 acknowledged that his eating pattern, lack of exercise, and overweight may have contributed to this current state of diabetes, he feels much more strongly that stress was the major reason.

"Blacks have a predisposition to diabetes due to our heredity, but it is the stress in our lives that is of most importance."

"Patient Informant No. 22 (African American male): *I really don't know what caused my diabetes. I have received a lot of explanations over the years, but I am still unsure of the actual cause."*

"Patient Informant No. 8 (African American female): *I'm not sure what caused my diabetes. I know that there is a family connection to diabetes and my weight has something to do with it, but I don't take all of it too seriously."*

When asked to assess her ability to follow the doctor's prescribed diabetic regimen, patient informant no. 8 stated:

"My sons and husband want their meals the way they normally have it. They don't want no unseasoned meals, so what am I supposed to do?"

"Patient Informant No. 4 (African American male): *I was really not shocked when I was diagnosed with diabetes simply because my father and aunt have diabetes and I knew it was a matter of time before I would develop it."*

"Diabetes is common among African Americans and this is due to our dietary eating pattern—fried foods and not enough vegetables."

Although patient informant no. 4 felt that it was a matter of time before he would develop diabetes, he is still unsure of the process and the reasons he developed type 2 diabetes. He came to the clinic only to find out what was wrong with his stomach. To his surprise, he was diagnosed with type 2 diabetes.

Stage 3: Quantitative Interviews and Analysis of the Semi-structured Questionnaire

Stage 3 consisted of testing and evaluating a culturally sensitive semi-structured questionnaire to be used in a clinical setting to assess the health beliefs and health care seeking pattern of the African American diabetes patients. A comparison sample of European Americans with similar duration of diabetes and similar age, sex, and socioeconomic status was also interviewed.

The quantitative data were gathered from the questionnaire and entered into the mainframe computers at Indiana University/Purdue

University Computer Center. The statistical package SPSS was used to analyze the data. The data analyses sought to determine the factors related to perceptions of diabetes, symptoms related to treatment for diabetes, health care seeking behavior, and adherence to the diabetic regimen. Standard parametric statistics such as t-test, Pearson correlations, and multiple regressions were used to support the findings.

The sociodemographics of this study's sample were as follows:

A.   Ethnic Background
    1.   African American (40%)
    2.   Euro-American (56%)
    3.   Other (4%)

B.   Gender
    1.   Males (68%)
    2.   Females (32%)

C.   Educational Background
    1.   High school education or equivalent (48%)
    2.   Less than a high school education (30%)
    3.   College education (22%)

D.   Total Sample = 25 patients *Research Findings: Quantitative Results*

The quantitative analyses found a number of significant differences between African American and European American diabetes patients in relation to their diabetic regimen. The significant differences were:

1.   African Americans (70%) were more likely than European Americans (35%) to agree that their diabetes is well controlled ($p = .02$).

2.   European Americans (100%) were more likely than African Americans (60%) to disagree with the statement, "I cannot understand what the doctor told me about my diet/medication/and diabetes" ($p = .05$).

3.   African Americans (50%) were less likely than European Americans (14%) to recognize diabetes-related symptoms ($p = .05$).

4.   European Americans (100%) were more likely than African Americans (80%) to believe that excess weight is related to diabetes ($p = .05$).

5.   African Americans (50%) were more likely than European Americans (14%) to seek care at the clinic for their diabetes (p = .05).

6.   African Americans (50%) were more likely than European Americans (7%) to join a support group for their diabetes (p = .03).

7.   European Americans (81%) were more likely than African Americans (20%) to know their blood sugar count when arriving for a scheduled visit to the Diabetes Clinic (p = .03).

Summary

In this two-year applied medical anthropology study, the cultural health beliefs and health care seeking pattern of African American diabetic patients significantly influenced individuals' degree of adherence to their diabetic regimen. The combination of the quantitative and the qualitative data indicates that African Americans experience uncertainty about their diabetic condition. In one respect, African Americans believed that they were well controlled and felt that they understood what the doctor told them about their diabetes. On the other hand, qualitative data (personal statements from patient informants) stated that there was a high degree of uncertainty about the cause of one's diabetes and how to treat it. In addition, African American diabetic patients tend not to be aware of the symptoms related to diabetes; tend not to know their blood sugar levels; and tend not to know the major factors associated with the development of diabetes.

The next question is: Why don't African American patients know more about their diabetes? As indicated from the quantitative data, the answer is that African Americans honestly believe that they have received enough information from health care professionals and friends to take control of their diabetes. Thus, it is not that the African American patient was not being told about his or her diabetic condition; rather, the lack of adherence to the diabetic regimen relates more to the lack of understanding between the two parties (patient and health care professional) when they discuss the patient's diabetic condition. Both parties felt that they understood each other, but in actuality they did not. African Americans were not aware of the direct relationship that overweight and obesity has with the development of type 2 diabetes. This lack of understanding results in the poor adherence to the diabetic regimen among African Americans.

Finally, my research study major findings are reflected in the comments made by the former president of the National Medical Association, Yvonnecris Smith Veal, in 1996. She stated that there are three basic reasons why diabetes continues to plague the African American community.

"First, there are the lifestyle and behavioral patterns associated with African Americans, such as poor eating habits, obesity, limited access to adequate medical care, and limited funds. African Americans in general tend to eat foods high in calories and loaded with saturated fats and sugar, along with having a sedentary lifestyle—all of which are contributing factors to overweight. Second, African Americans have a history of preparing foods with lard and other heavy oils. This type of food preparation, along with the inability to obtain a balanced diet, contributes to the risk factors associated with diabetes. Third, African Americans need more options to choose dietary diabetic regimens that fit the preferences for certain foods and eating practices among all segments of the African American population." (Veal 1996: 203)

The Michigan Example: African American Women Healthy Lifestyles Initiative

Another example of the effects of obesity in the African American community originates from the state of Michigan. In 1991, Michigan was one of four states with obesity rates higher than the rest of the nation. This trend has persisted over time, as the rate of obesity in Michigan has remained consistently high in comparison to the rest of the United States. Michigan behavioral risk database (BRFSS) indicated that in 2001 almost one-quarter of adults (24.7%) were obese, more than double the rate in 1987 (12.2%) (Michigan Department of Community Health 2002: 2).

Rates of obesity among African Americans, especially women, were particularly high compared with other population groups. In 1999, 35.9% of African American women were obese, an increase of 146% compared with 1987 (Michigan Department of Community Health 2002: 4).

In an effort to stop this increasing trend of obesity in Michigan and particularly among African American women, the Michigan Department of Community Health (MDCH) applied for and received a grant from the Centers for Disease Control and Prevention to fund the development of a state plan to prevent and control overweight and obesity in a focused population through healthy eating and physical activity. The effort, named the *Healthy Lifestyle Initiative,* convened a 52-member Statewide Planning Committee to guide the production of a focused state plan to combat overweight and obesity. The committee members represented organizations with expertise in physical activity, healthy eating, minority issues, research, communications, and community development (Michigan Department of Community Health 2002: 6).

The committee divided into three subcommittees to explore specific issues such as behavior, policy, environment, and communications. Over six months, with staff help from the Michigan Department of Community Health, the committee completed the following:

- Determined that African American women, the highest risk segment, should be the priority population addressed in the strategic plan.

- Reviewed existing data and literature and offered expert information about factors contributing to overweight and obesity in this population.

- Produced an inventory of programs and services related to physical activity, healthy eating, and/or obesity focused on Michigan counties with the highest percentage of African American residents.

- Identified the main barriers to African American women being active and eating well.

- Developed and prioritized strategies to facilitate healthy eating and physical activity.

- Provided recommendations for creation of a state plan. (Michigan Department of Community Health 2002: 7)

With regard to the specific factors contributing to overweight and obesity in African American women in Michigan, the committee and the Michigan Department of Community Health found that:

1. They were not communicating effectively with African American women regarding physical activity and healthy eating.

2. The living environment of many African American women in Michigan is not supportive of physical activity and healthy eating.

3. It is perceived that health care providers are not effectively addressing the needs of African American women in regard to physical activity, healthy eating, and overweight/obesity.

4. Personal characteristics and concerns can contribute to physical inactivity and unhealthy eating.

5. Cultural and social issues can impact adoption of healthy behaviors. (Michigan Department of Community Health 2002: 11–14)

In summary, the committee made the following recommendations for the state to implement in order to reduce the rate of overweight and obesity in the African American communities throughout the state of Michigan:

1. **Communications and Education:** Contribute to an atmosphere supportive of a healthy lifestyle by providing positive messages and information about nutrition, physical activity, and healthy weight-loss strategies to African American women.

2. **Supportive Communities:** Facilitate social, policy, and environmental changes to ensure that communities improve physical activity and healthy eating environments.

3. **Programs:** Provide culturally appropriate opportunities to learn how to be active, eat healthfully, and achieve/maintain a healthy weight.

4. **Health Care Providers/Systems:** Increase the percentage of health care providers counseling African American female patients in a culturally sensitive manner on overweight/obesity.

5. **Surveillance, Epidemiology, and Evaluation:** Establish methods and systems to gather and disseminate data and monitor trends for overweight/obesity, healthy eating, and physical activity specifically for African American women.

6. **Resources and Infrastructure:** Increase resources and expand infrastructure for obesity prevention and control.

7. **Research:** Using a social marketing framework, implement and evaluate pilot project(s) for the priority population that impact(s) overweight/obesity through physical activity and healthy eating. (Michigan Department of Community Health 2002: 8–10)

This Michigan example not only typifies many African American women's problems with overweight and obesity but also shows how state government initiatives attempt to reduce the disparity of overweight and obesity in the African American community. Whether Michigan's Community Health Department made an impact with this African American women's overweight and obesity initiative or not, it is significant to note that there have been comprehensive and culturally competent weight-loss programs developed for African American communities in the United States. Because this is the case, why haven't these comprehensive and culturally competent weight-loss programs been effective?

A Recent Study on Weight-Loss Experiences Among African American Women

In one of the most recent studies on obesity among African American women, researchers discovered that certain cultural factors hindered African American women in adhering to their weight-loss program (Davis et al. 2005). In this study, Dr. Esa Davis and her colleagues investigated the racial and socioeconomic factors that impacted weight management practices among obese women. Their study's results not only confirmed the results of other related studies but also helped to highlight even more significantly the impact on how certain aspects of African American culture may cause African Americans to fail in weight-management programs.

The Davis et al. (2005) study involved 27 obese African American and white women aged 20 to 65 years who worked for the same Maryland employer in a 90-minute discussion on their past and current experiences with weight-loss practices and how their race, social class, and educational level affected personal weight-management efforts. Four focus group sessions were conducted to collect the data from the sampled group of African American and white women.

Audiotapes were transcribed verbatim, and participants' names were replaced with codes. Two investigators independently read each transcript in its entirety and marked distinct comments that could be categorized into themes. A third investigator adjudicated differences in theme assignment between the first reviewers. Themes and comments underwent independent second review for relevancy and consistency by two other investigators, this process resulted in consolidation of some themes and separation of others into subthemes (Davis et al. 2005: 1539).

The findings from the focus group sessions of African American and white women resulted in six major themes. The themes were as follows:

1.   Failure of weight maintenance
2.   Psychological and spiritual approaches
3.   Family influence and societal expectations
4.   African American subculture hinders weight management
5.   Affordability concerns limit weight management
6.   Racial differences in ideal weight-loss methods

For the first theme, "Failure of weight maintenance," Davis et al. (2005) found that all of the women attempted weight loss with various methods, including diet, diet pills, exercise, and alternative methods such as hypnosis and fasting. Most women preferred weight-loss methods that incorporated a weight-maintenance focus to prevent them from weight cycling and relapse.

In particular, African American women stated the following:

"The one thing I find with the (weight loss) programs is, it's good to help you lose weight, but the problem is they really don't teach you how to maintain." (Davis et al. 2005: 1541)

For the second theme, "Psychological and spiritual approaches," Davis et al. (2005) found that the inability to sustain weight loss over a long period fueled significant negative emotions, including pain, desperation, frustration, and boredom among all the women. Women in all four groups wanted their emotional and psychological concerns to be remediated in weight-management programs. African American women preferred to have these concerns remediated through spiritual means.

Specifically, African American women stated the following:

> *"This is about the biggest struggle I have in my life—weight loss ... I tend to pray a lot and fast a lot. When I want changes in my life, that's what changes it."*

> *"I think for me the spiritual piece is very important. Without it, any weight-loss program is not gonna work. You need a dual program."* (Davis et al. 2005: 1541)

For the third theme, "Family influences and societal expectations," Davis et al. (2005) found that women believed that their negative feelings about weight management and being overweight stemmed from the influence of their family of origin and from societal standards learned from childhood. Some African American women described being teased about being overweight, but others recalled being pressured by family members to accept being overweight. Both African American and white women believed that the societal expectations of thinness were difficult for them to achieve.

Specifically, African American women stated the following:

> *"For most of my life, through various sources of input, I've had a negative body image ... They (my grandparents) would tease me: 'You're fat,' 'You're never going to be anybody if you're fat' and then that would just make me feel bad about myself."*

> *"One thing was always told to me: 'We're a big-boned family. Child, you are always gonna be big. Don't worry about it. You will never be small because it's just the way this family is built.'"* (Davis et al. 2005: 1541)

For the fourth theme, "African American subculture hinders weight management," Davis et al. (2005) found that American cultural support of sedentary lifestyles, excessive food availability, and media influences appeared to make weight loss challenging for all four groups. However, African American women in both SES (socioeconomic status) groups identified African American cultural influences, including settings (e.g., church, sorority meetings); cultural food types (e.g., collard greens, fried chicken), preparation, and abundance; and beliefs and expectations about food (e.g., focus on food in social gatherings) that further complicated successful weight management.

Specifically, African American women stated the following:

"It's eating and cooking and sharing, that's a Black thing, particularly in the churches."

"Church is our life, it's our outlet. Where the world may go to the clubs and go to bars, food is our outlet. If you want people to come out, you better tell them there's going to be some food."

"One of our (African American women) downfalls is cultural. Yes, the Southern cooking. I'll start with collard greens and put in fat meat, hog maws or ham hocks, in there." (Davis et al. 2005: 1541)

For the fifth theme, "Affordability concerns limit weight management efforts," Davis et al. (2005) found that all groups discussed the expense of weight-loss practices, but the lower SES groups expressed a higher level of cost concern; they believed that affordability limited their weight-management efforts despite their desire to lose weight.

African American women stated the following:

"If you are not consistent in being there (Weight Watchers program), you may not always have $8 at that moment, I mean I don't always have (it), or it has to go to something else at that time."

"You know, 3 boxes of macaroni and cheese for a dollar as opposed to buying chicken breasts that are, you know 10 bucks, if you get 2 of them." (Davis et al. 2005: 1541)

For the final theme, "Racial differences in ideal weight-loss methods," Davis et al. (2005) found that white women emphasized physical activity and did not mention food characteristics, whereas African American women emphasized food characteristics such as taste, texture, and types in their ideal weight-loss method and made no references to physical activity.

An African American woman stated the following:

"Food that tastes good as opposed to bland, flavorless food, food with various textures, and what have you." (Davis et al. 2005: 1541)

Overall, Davis et al. (2005) study's findings have several specific implications for weight-management interventions. First, the African American indicated that short-term weight loss is achievable, yet maintaining weight loss is difficult. Future intervention should emphasize weight-maintenance strategies to prevent weight cycling and relapse. Because spirituality appears important to African American women, programs targeting this population might incorporate spiritual messages and methods. Participants' reports of the influence of negative family input during childhood on weight perceptions suggest that health professionals should encourage adults to provide positive messages to children regarding eating patterns, food selection, and body weight (Davis et al. 2005: 1542).

In addition, Davis et al. (2005) state that the racial differences in ideal weight-loss method components identified in this study should prompt further investigation into factors such as attention to taste and cultural appropriateness of food and hindrances to physical activity for African American women. Finally, creative strategies that educate low SES women on cost-effective ways to eat healthy and engage in physical activity are needed (Davis et al. 2005: 1542).

Conclusion

The facts are the facts. Just like a majority of Americans, African Americans are becoming more and more overweight and obese than ever before. Like a majority of Americans, African Americans are also suffering from the consequences of overweight and obesity such as heart attacks, strokes, and type 2 diabetes at an earlier age. Too many African Americans are losing their lives due to overweight and obesity. Finally, like a majority of Americans, African Americans have embraced this *cultural and societal pattern* that being bigger and fat is okay.

Well, let me make it perfectly clear that I have nothing against individuals who choose to be big and fat. We, as African Americans, have always embraced individuals of varying body types and varying body sizes (big, large, small, skinny, tall, and short). The fact that mainstream society is steadily incorporating African American physical (fuller and shapely figures) and cultural (Spoken Soul, clothing, hair styles, and music) attributes into their "societal standard" paradigm is actually a compliment.

Yet I do want those who choose to be overweight (and there are many) to be healthy and have a quality of life that they deserve. That's one of the major reasons I wrote this book.

Another reason I wrote this book is to provide myself and others a strategy that happens to be *culturally based* and *culturally designed* to fit our particular African American perspectives on health, fitness, dieting, food, and exercise. I believe this African American perspective is desperately needed today because what we are talking about now is our survival, and we have no more time to waste.

Therefore, instead of blaming our culture, which a lot of people do when things do not go right in the African American community, I have used various aspects of our culture in helping us to address and solve many of the issues surrounding overweight and obesity in our diverse communities. That's why this book examines body image, body type, and body build from the African American perspective. That's why this book examines food practices and the cultural meaning of *soul food* from the African American perspective. That's why this book examines physical fitness and exercise from the African American perspective. Finally, that's why this book places dieting, health, and fitness in an African American cultural framework.

By taking this *cultural approach*, we can collectively work together in not only understanding comprehensively this critical health issue but also in developing a new cultural health and fitness program that works for you and many others who share your cultural perspective on health and fitness. If you feel the way that I do, then encourage others such as your sister, brother, uncle, aunt, cousin, grandma, granddad, children, and family friends to take this *cultural health and physical fitness* challenge with you.

So go ahead and try all the fancy and trendy diet and fitness programs that are currently out there in the market. After you've tried them and realize that they are really not talking or relating to you as an African American, then come back and give the New Black Cultural Diet™ a chance. You won't regret it!

Postevaluation Questions

1. How do health professionals begin to change the perspective of what constitutes "overweight" in the African American community?

    Health professionals can begin to change the perspective of what constitutes overweight in the African American community by first acknowledging the positive steps that an individual African American took in recognizing that he or she may be overweight. Once the health professionals approach the African American patient in a positive manner, then more constructive dialogue can occur that will slowly challenge and change the perspective of what constitutes overweight for the individual African American.

2. Should health professionals challenge African Americans' approach to health, diet, and fitness?

    Health professionals should cautiously challenge African Americans' approach to health, diet, and physical fitness in a culturally appropriate manner that takes into consideration an African American's traditional beliefs about health, diet, and physical fitness.

3.   How can African Americans get health professionals to better understand how they view overweight and obesity?

African Americans can get health professionals to better understand how they view overweight and obesity by starting to talk more about how they perceive healthy and nonhealthy behavioral pattern and lifestyle issues. Once individual African Americans begin this dialogue with their health providers about these basic issues, then the health provider can begin to develop a dietary and physical fitness maintenance program that best fits the individual African American patient.

References

Bailey, E. 2002. *Medical anthropology and African American health.* Westport, CT: Bergin and Garvey.

Davis, E., Clark, J., Carrese, J., Gary, T., and Cooper, L. 2005. Racial and socioeconomic differences in the weight-loss experiences of obese women. *American Journal of Public Health* 95(9):1539–1543.

Michigan Department of Community Health. 2002. *An epidemic of overweight and obesity in Michigan's African American women: A report of the healthy lifestyles initiative.* Lansing, Michigan: Michigan Department of Health. Available at http://www.michigan.gov/documents/ AAObesityreportc_89887 _7.pdf.

Mitchell, T. 2002. Keep moving toward the lite. *USA Weekend.* November 15–17:6–11.

National Institute of Diabetes and Digestive and Kidney Disorders (NIDDK). 2005. Diabetes overview. Available at http://diabetes.niddk.nih.gov/dm/pubs/overview/index.htm.

Satcher, D. 2001. Overweight and obesity threatens U.S. health gains. U.S. Department of Health and Human Services Press Release. Thursday, December 31, 2001. Available at http://www.surgeongeneral.gov/news/pressreleases/pr_obesity.htm.

Veal, Y. 1996. African Americans and diabetes: Reasons, rationale, and research. *Journal of the National Medical Association* 88:203–204.

Overweight and Obesity Among African Americans

2

Critical Thinking Questions

1. Why are African Americans not aware of their overweight and obesity statistics?
2. Should African Americans be concerned about the national data regarding their overweight and obesity statistics?
3. What are the major contributing factors for the higher prevalence of overweight and obesity among African Americans?
4. What can U.S. citizens do to change this pattern of increased overweight and obesity?

Introduction

Ironically, during a time when the amount of research activity, knowledge, and interest in obesity among the medical community, as well as the level of public attention to the issues of weight, diet, and exercise have never been greater, the epidemic of overweight and obesity continues virtually unchallenged and is misunderstood by the medical community and the public with no sight of reversal (Fontanarosa 2002). In fact, the basis of this entire health care problem—overweight and obesity—is not well understood and defined.

Overweight is defined as excessive weight for a given height and stature. *Obesity* is defined as an excessive amount of adipose tissue in the body (Gillum 1987: 866).

According to the National Institutes of Health (NIH), National Heart, Lung, and Blood Institute (NHLBI), *overweight* is defined as a body mass index (BMI) of 25 to 29.9 kg/m^2 and *obesity* as a BMI of $\geq$30 kg/m^2. However, overweight and obesity are not mutually exclusive, as obese persons are also overweight. A BMI of 30 is about 30 lb overweight and equivalent to 221 lb in a 6' 0" person and to 186 lb in one 5' 6" (NHLBI 1998).

Yet are these definitions accepted or known by the community and, most importantly, are these definitions considered important to the community? The following health statistics on overweight and obesity among African Americans, the general U.S. population, and U.S. children will give you some evidence as to whether Americans consider these definitions important or not.

Overweight and Obesity Among African Americans: The Facts

As indicated in the previous discussion about overweight and obesity, the proportion of Americans who are overweight and obese has increased dramatically within the past two decades. The fact that increases in overweight and obesity cuts across all ages, racial and ethnic groups, and both genders indicates that this health-care problem should be a national priority.

Previous Data

The prevalence rates for African Americans have also continued to soar during the past decades. Specifically, McTigue, Garrett, and Popkin (2002), in an article entitled "The Natural History of the Development of Obesity in a Cohort of Young U.S. Adults Between 1981 and 1998" in the *Annals of Internal Medicine,* found that obesity onset was 2.1 times faster for black women and 1.5 times faster for Hispanic women than for white women. For men, they found both black men and white showing similar rates of obesity onset at the transition into adulthood, but obesity developed more rapidly in black men after approximately age 28 years. Studies such as Gillum (1987), Burke et al. (1992), Shavers, V., and Shankar, S., (2002); U.S. Department of Health and Human Services (1997) and the U.S. Surgeon General (Satcher 2001) found similar results.

McTigue, Garrett, and Popkin's (2002) study sample of 9,179 born between 1957 and 1964 and followed for two decades included only persons who reported that the ethnicity with which they most closely identified was Hispanic, black, or white (or European origin). They contend that in their sample, black women and Hispanic men were at highest risk for obesity. Efforts to prevent or treat obesity in black men should take into consideration the delay in elevated risk in this group until late in the third decade of life. Although they cannot assess the cause of such differences in their study, it is important to note that race or ethnicity and sex are likely surrogates, totally or in part, for other factors such as dietary and exercise standards, income, education, and parity. Finally, McTigue, Garrett, and Popkin (2002: 863) strongly suggest that further examination is essential if we are to understand underlying culture-specific contributors to obesity.

Current Data

According to data from the Centers for Disease Control and Prevention's National Health Interview Survey, black adults (30.4%) were considerably more likely than white adults (20.8%) to be obese. In this report, entitled "Health Behaviors of Adults: United States, 1999–2001," researchers found that black men (24.9%) were significantly less likely than black women (34.9%) to be obese. Additionally, among black adults and Native Hawaiian or other Pacific Islander adults, prevalence of overweight was about the same for men as for women (Centers for Disease Control and Prevention 2004).

The statistical trend showing that African Americans are experiencing higher prevalence of overweight and obesity is also illustrated in several other national studies (Gordon-Larsen, Adair, and Popkin 2003; Daniels et al. 2005; National Center for Health Statistics 1997). For example, in a survey of 4,115 adult men and women in 1999 and 2000, data from the National Health and Nutrition Examination Survey (NHANES) showed that among women, obesity and overweight prevalences were highest among non-Hispanic black women. More than half of non-Hispanic black women aged 40 years or older were obese and more than 80% were overweight (Flegal et al. 2002).

Overweight and Obesity in America: The Facts

So how prevalent is obesity among Americans? According to the Centers for Disease Control and Prevention, for the first time in history, there are more overweight and obese people in the nation than people of normal weight. In a report entitled "Prevalence of Overweight and Obesity Among Adults: United States, 1999," initial results from the 1999 National Health and Nutrition Examination Survey, using measured heights and weights, indicate that an estimated 61 percent of U.S. adults are either overweight or obese (Centers for Disease Control and Prevention 1999).

The impact of overweight and obesity on the health status of Americans is such an important topic that the former U.S. Surgeon General, Dr. David Satcher, organized an investigation of this health issue and completed a report entitled "The Surgeon General's Call to Action to Prevent and Decrease Overweight and Obesity." Dr. Satcher's report outlined strategies that communities can use in helping to address the problems. Those options include requiring physical education at all school grades, providing more healthy food options on school campuses, and providing safe and accessible recreational facilities for residents of all ages. If we do not implement these strategies, then Dr. Satcher believes that "overweight and obesity may soon cause as much preventable disease and death as cigarette smoking."

This is a powerful statement and a very significant report from the former Surgeon General emphasizing that our country needs to take action now and not think that this problem will go away. Data has shown that this problem is getting bigger and bigger every year and that U.S. citizens are suffering from more overweight- and obesity-related health problems than ever before (Centers for Disease Control and Prevention 2002a and 2002b). Moreover, there are other national studies finally recognizing this epidemic.

In a landmark evaluation of data collected from all states that participated in the Behavioral Risk Factor Surveillance System (BRFSS) study, a study conducted from 1991 to 1998 among adults aged 18 years or older, Mokdad et al. (1999) found that the prevalence of obesity increased from 12.0 percent in 1991 to 17.9 percent in 1998. Obesity increased in men and women and across all sociodemographic groups with the highest increase among the youngest ages and higher education levels (Mokdad et al. 1999: 1520).

Among ethnic minority groups, the prevalence of obesity among blacks increased from 19 percent in 1991 to 27 percent in 1998. This is a 39 percent increase. Among Hispanics, the prevalence of obesity increased from 12 percent in 1991 to 21 percent in 1998. This is an 80 percent increase (Mokdad et al. 1999: 1520).

Interestingly, a paper by Flores et al. (2002) in the *Journal of the American Medical Association*, "The Health of Latino Children: Urgent Priorities, Unanswered Questions, and a Research Agenda," supports this data on Hispanics' increased obesity rates. In fact, they state that Latino boys are the most overweight and Latina girls the second most overweight racial/ethnic groups of U.S. children. Flores et al. (2002) emphasize that more research is needed to determine why Latino children have such high risks of obesity and diabetes and what preventive interventions are most effective (Flores et al. 2002: 86).

Additional data from Mokdad's article in the *Journal of the American Medical Association,* entitled "The Spread of the Obesity Epidemic in the United States, 1991–1998," include:

- In 1991, 4 of the 45 participating states had obesity rates of 15 percent or higher. By 1998, 37 states had rates higher than 15 percent.

- In 1991, the level of leisure-time physical activity was 29.7 percent inactive, 28.4 percent irregularly active, 33.2 percent regular not intense, and 8.7 percent regular intense. In 1998, they were 28.6 percent inactive, 28.2 percent irregularly active, 29.6 percent regular not intense, and 13.6 percent regular intense.

In general, Mokdad et al. (1999) state that these data show that obesity increased in every state, in both sexes, and across all age groups, races, educational levels, and smoking statuses. They contend that this rapid increase in obesity in all segments of the population and regions of the country implies that there have been sweeping changes in U.S. society that are contributing to weight gain by fostering energy intake imbalance. Furthermore, they feel that when focusing on the challenge of stopping the obesity epidemic and the profound negative health consequences of obesity, it is important to increase the awareness and involvement of health professionals in dealing with the epidemic (Mokdad et al. 1999: 1521).

So is there a direct relationship between obesity and certain types of chronic diseases? According to the National Center for Chronic Disease Prevention and Health Promotion at the Centers for Disease Control and Prevention, the increasing prevalence of obesity is a major public health concern because obesity is associated with several chronic diseases such as heart disease, cancer, stroke, and diabetes (Mokdad et al. 1999). In fact, excess weight is associated with an increased incidence of cardiovascular disease, type 2 diabetes mellitus (DM), hypertension, stroke, dyslipidemia, osteoarthritis, and some cancers (Burton et al. 1985; Allison et al. 1999; Must et al. 1999).

Perhaps one of the most startling reports emphasizing the damaging effects of overweight and obesity on Americans came from a special report in the *New England Journal of Medicine* (Olshansky et al. 2005). In the article, "A Potential Decline in Life Expectancy in the United States in the 21st Century," researchers stipulated that if the prevalence of obesity continues to rise, especially at younger ages, the negative effect on health and longevity in the coming decades could be much worse.

In fact, the researchers contend that:

"Unless effective population-level interventions to reduce obesity are developed, the steady rise in life expectancy observed in the modern era may soon come to an end and the youth of today may, on average, live less healthy and possibly even

shorter lives than their parents. The health and life expectancy of minority populations may be hit hardest by obesity, because within these subgroups, access to health care is limited and childhood and adult obesity has increased the fastest. In fact, if the negative effect of obesity on life expectancy continues to worsen, and current trends in prevalence suggest it will, then gains in health and longevity that have taken decades to achieve may be quickly reversed." (Olshansky et al. 2005: 1143)

Now that we have supportive data to link obesity and overweight with certain types of chronic diseases, what is the next step for our health care system? It is time not only to address the problem of obesity and overweight in our society but also to develop national, state, and local programs that can make a significant impact on this serious health-care issue. Without concerted initiatives to prevent and treat overweight in adults and now in children, the health care system will increasingly be overwhelmed with individuals who require treatment for obesity-related health conditions (Must et al. 1999: 1529).

Overweight and Obesity in Children: The Facts

In 2005, Robert Eckel, president-elect of the American Heart Association, joined former President Bill Clinton and Arkansas Governor Mike Huckabee in a new initiative sponsored by the American Heart Association, the Robert Wood Johnson Foundation, and the William J. Clinton Foundation to fight childhood obesity. Eckel stated that:

> *"The rate has doubled in children and tripled in teens in the last 25 years."* (CBS2 News 2005; Daniels et al. 2005)

This new initiative, launched at an event at New York City's Public School 128, aims to target several areas that the group hopes will spark change and slow the increasing rates of childhood obesity in the United States and encourage healthier lifestyles for young people. The effort will focus on the following areas:

- **Industry:** Working with the food and restaurant industry to improve the quality of offerings and to develop marketing and promotion strategies to support environmental change within the industry; convening key industry players in consumer packaged food, food service, and exercise/fitness to develop healthier eating and more exercise.

- **Schools and Community Groups:** Increasing physical activity and improving nutrition in schools across the nation; providing standards for schools to improve the food served in cafeterias and vending machines; improving opportunities for enhanced physical activity both in school and after school.

- **Community Mobilization:** Creating a campaign to engage kids in taking steps to make healthy lifestyle choices; providing tools and information to help parents incorporate heart-healthy activities into family routines; creating tools and providing opportunities for health-care providers to better recognize, prevent, and treat obesity in children.

- **Media:** Exploring opportunities to work with the media to encourage healthier lifestyles for young people; activities will include using role models to promote heart-healthy lifestyles among youth.

According to Eckel, "We need to go right to the source and bring kids—all kids—into the equation. This is not just about kids who are already overweight or obese. This is about helping kids of all shapes and sizes to control their health and to create lifelong habits that emphasize balance, better nutrition and increased activity." (Clinton Foundation Organization 2005).

In 2002, the National Institutes of Health, Office of Research on Women's Health sponsored a seminar entitled "Promoting Healthy Lives: Diet, Fat & Cholesterol." The event featured three experts to present the facts and, perhaps more importantly, refute the innumerable myths that swirl around these topics. Dr. Frank Sacks, a professor of cardiovascular disease prevention at Harvard School of Public Health, Dr. Gary Foster, clinical director of the Weight and Eating Disorders Program at the University of Pennsylvania School of Medicine, and Dr. Pamela Peeke, a former NIH senior research fellow and an internationally recognized expert on nutrition and stress, tackled the tough questions of what to eat (Garnett 2002).

According to Dr. Peeke (2002), "Americans are eating potentially too much of certain fats, and the forms of fat we're eating and the way those fats are processed—that's really where the topic should begin." Moreover she stated, "the saddest part about this is what is happening to the children."

"One out of four is quite overweight and obesity is rising, as are the consequences. Children with type 2 diabetes are much more prevalent. This used to be an old person's disease. We're

now diagnosing this at ages 7, 10, 15. The incidence of type 2
diabetes between ages 30 and 40 has increased 70 percent."

Is this in fact the truth? Are overweight and obesity having a tremendous effect among children in the United States? Because overweight youths may become overweight adults and overweight adults are at increased risk for adverse health outcomes, overweight in childhood is gaining increasing recognition as an important public health concern. If so, then what do the statistics tell us?

According to the National Health and Nutrition Examination Surveys from 1963 to 1991, which consisted of 14,000 youths aged 6 through 17 years, the prevalence of overweight for children and adolescents was 22 percent. Among girls in both age groups (aged 6 through 11 years and 12 through 17 years), non-Hispanic blacks had the highest prevalence of overweight and non-Hispanic whites had the lowest prevalence. For boys aged 6 through 11 years, non-Hispanic whites had the lowest prevalence of overweight, whereas for boys aged 12 through 17 years, non-Hispanic blacks had the lowest prevalence (Troiano et al. 1995: 1086).

Although some overweight youths will lose their excess weight as they mature and develop, Troiano et al. (1995) contend that it is likely that many will go on to become overweight adults. The current prevalence of overweight among youths and the likelihood of continued, if not additional, high prevalence as these youths age implies increased need for treatment of morbidities associated with overweight in the near and distant future.

Moreover, increases in overweight may be attributable to more than changes in the behavior of individuals. From a population perspective, the trends observed for all age groups in the United States and in many other societies worldwide suggest social and environmental factors that are affecting many individuals similarly (Ogden, C., Flegal, K., Carroll, M., and Johnson, C. 2002; Troiano and Flegal 1998: 503).

After Troiano and colleagues' study, additional studies on the prevalence of childhood overweight and obesity continued. For example, an article entitled "Epidemic Increase in Childhood Overweight, 1986–1998" in the *Journal of the American Medical Association* (Strauss and Pollack 2001) concluded that childhood overweight continues to increase rapidly in the United States. Specifically, Strauss and Pollack (2001) examined the data from the National Longitudinal Survey of Youth, a prospective cohort study conducted from 1986 to 1998 among 8,270 children aged 4 to 12 years, as well as a supplemental sample of Hispanics, African Americans, and poor whites, and found that overweight increased significantly and steadily among African American, Hispanic, and white children.

By 1998, overweight prevalence had increased by more than 120 percent among African Americans and Hispanics and by more than 50 percent among whites. By 1998, 21.5 percent of African American children and 21.8 percent of Hispanic children were overweight. In contrast, 12.3 percent of white children were overweight (Strauss and Pollack 2001: 2846).

Additionally, large differences in overweight prevalence emerged between groups over the study period. For instance, 1986 overweight prevalence was virtually identical among upper-income white girls and among lower-income African American and Hispanic boys (6.6% vs. 6.5%, p = .95). Yet by 1998, overweight prevalence had increased only slightly to 8.7 percent among upper-income white girls, whereas overweight prevalence had increased to 27.4 percent among lower-income African American and Hispanic boys (Strauss and Pollack 2001: 2846).

Strauss and Pollack (2001) conclude from their analyses that the prevalence of childhood overweight is rapidly increasing, with the sharpest observed increases among boys, African Americans, Hispanics, and those living in Southern states. By 1998, more than 21 percent of African American and Hispanic children were classified as overweight. These race/ethnic trend disparities remained large and statistically significant after controlling for family income and other cofounders. They suggest that childhood overweight is prevalent because it arises from deeply rooted behaviors and from social practices that are hardly confined to children. Given the profound consequences of childhood inactivity, poor nutrition, and overweight through the life span, urgency is warranted in responding to this epidemic (Strauss and Pollack 2001: 2848).

In 2001, the Surgeon General's office recognized this epidemic among children and concurred with earlier studies. Former Surgeon General, Dr. David Satcher, released data on childhood overweight in the report entitled "The Surgeon General's Call to Action to Prevent and Decrease Overweight and Obesity," and stated the following key points:

- In 1991, 13 percent of children aged 6 to 11 years and 14 percent of adolescents aged 12 to 19 years in the United States were overweight. This prevalence has nearly tripled for adolescents in the past two decades.

- Risk factors for heart disease, such as high cholesterol and high blood pressure, occur with increased frequency in overweight children and adolescents compared with children with a healthy weight.

- Type 2 diabetes, previously considered an adult disease, has increased dramatically in children and adolescents.

Overweight and obesity are closely linked to type 2 diabetes.

- Overweight adolescents have a 70 percent chance of becoming overweight or obese adults. This increases to 80 percent if one or both parents are overweight or obese. Overweight or obese adults are at risk for a number of health problems including heart disease, type 2 diabetes, high blood pressure, and some forms of cancer.

- The most immediate consequences of overweight as perceived by the children themselves is social discrimination. This is associated with poor self-esteem and depression (Satcher 2001).

If this is not enough evidence about childhood overweight and obesity, then I do not know what is.

To examine more closely the issues of overweight and obesity among adolescents, Thompson and Story (2003) conducted focus groups with urban, African American caretakers of preschool children. The purpose of this study was to elicit the perceptions regarding obesity in their community, with an emphasis on childhood obesity. These purposes were:

1. How did the participants define obesity?

2. Did the participants perceive obesity, especially in childhood, to be a problem?

3. How did the participants judge whether a child was overweight or obese?

4. How did the participants define healthy eating patterns for themselves and for their children?

5. What were the participants' ideas about the prevalence and causes of overweight in their community?

6. What was the lifestyle information such as usual eating and child-feeding patterns?

7. What were the perceptions that could be elicited of relationships among weight, health, diet, and other health-related behaviors?

8. Were the characteristics of information, support, and interventions viewed by target population members as welcome and helpful in preventing or ameliorating obesity? (Thompson and Story 2003: 29)

A convenience sample of 34 participants, 28 women and 6 men, was recruited by the administrators of a Head Start center located in the designated community, a neighborhood in the inner-city of a medium-sized city located in the Mid-Atlantic region. The three focus groups had 13, 11, and 10 participants, respectively. All participants were African American, ranging in age from 18 to the late fifties (Thompson and Story 2003: 29).

The three focus groups were facilitated by one of two trained and experienced moderators who used a questioning guide and were assisted by a member of the research team. One moderator was a European American female in her twenties and the other an African American female in her thirties.

Moderators used a questioning guide that was designed for two purposes: (1) to gain a greater understanding of participants' insiders' views of obesity among children and adults in their community; and (2) to elicit information on themes that the literature suggests might be important for designing an effective obesity-prevention intervention for the target population (Thompson and Story 2003: 29).

Several themes emerged from the focus groups. First, participants indicated that obesity connoted a very extreme condition to them. According to their participants, an obese person would have serious health problems and would not be able to function normally due to weight. Several participants vehemently expressed that they did not consider classification as overweight or obese using height-and-weight charts to be valid for them personally. They considered these charts to be biased, in part due to factors associated with their ethnicity and frame size. For example, participants stated the following:

> "I would define it as body weight maybe two to three times their normal weight ... with health ailment, who consistently like to eat. They're never full, that type."

> "OK, as far as obesity ... like, I had a cousin that ... was really, really overweight. He was a really heavy person. He didn't let his weight stop him from doing the things he wanted to do." (Thompson and Story 2003: 31)

Second, overweight as defined by height and weight charts was not viewed as a problem unless weight-related health problems were already present and serious. Although one person did associate obesity with poor health outcomes, no one spoke in terms of increased risk of developing health conditions in the future as a common consequence of overweight. Participants seemed to feel that having a large body size is normal for some people and how they "should" be, based on familial and ethnic patterns, which may be reflected in being active and not suffering from weight-related limitations or ailments. For example, participants also stated the following:

"You know, you have body frames, and you have cultures that are different, where bones play a big structure. My family, we … have hips, thighs, that type of thing. And where does that come into effect? How could you relate that because I'm 5'7? and I'm supposed to be quote, unquote, by these statistics, maybe 140. I'm not 140, and that's considering me as obese." (Thompson and Story 2003: 31)

Third, pediatricians and nutritionists were viewed as the experts who could diagnose and treat childrens' weight problems that had not responded to commonsense measures used within the family. Although participants truly believed that height-and-weight charts for adults were ethnically biased and not valid, they did state that pediatricians were able to diagnose overweight in a child. The type of practical information given by nutritionists, such as the amount of sugar in juice drinks or the number of calories in buttered microwave popcorn, was identified as powerful and useful and was reported to have an effect on subsequent food choices. Participants stated:

"Believe me, once you go to that nutritionist, and she shows you how much sugar is in the stuff that you eat, it will scare the life out of you, and … it will make you start reading those labels."

"Pediatricians need to get on top of the weight gain. It should start getting the child developed, like, frequent shots and so forth; they can start monitoring them." (Thompson and Story 2003: 31)

Finally, participants shared thoughts on the kinds of information, advice, strategies, or interventions they perceived as being helpful in preventing or ameliorating children's problems with overweight. They shared tips on strategies that had worked in their experience with improving children's eating habits or helping them lose extra weight. In discussing methods of increasing physical activity, participants emphasized the importance of having fun; dancing on a machine with computerized music was a form of play that children were reported to embrace enthusiastically. Participants felt that parents needed to be educated but that teaching strategies should not be dry or didactic. Instead, teaching strategies that participants consider the best are those that are interactive, hands-on, behaviorally based, and have direct application to learners' daily dietary decisions. Participants stated:

"They had an excellent class a couple of years ago where they actually gave you a certain amount of money to go out and

purchase food, and the nutritionist came, and the parents pre-pared foods. Some hands-on kinds of things, so it wasn't just sending you literature home and saying, 'Read it.' And they actually took them to the market, and helped them read labels." (Thompson and Story 2003: 32)

In conclusion, Thompson and Story's (2003) research suggests that nurses, pediatricians, and other health-care professionals should clearly and energetically communicate concern over young children's weight to mothers and other caretakers at an early date. Based on comments expressed in these focus groups, parents believe health professionals should treat the problem seriously and that parents should receive clear information and support for addressing weight problems in young children.

Moreover, one lesson to be drawn from this research is that the health education field needs to learn more about the ways various cultural, ethnic, and social groups experience language, labels, and other terminology commonly used in the field. Avoidance of terms found objectionable by target population members will make it easier for nurses and other health educators to form and maintain positive connections with patients and increase the likelihood that health-behavior messages will be heard, accepted, and acted upon. Therefore, we need research that explores the language and content of messages that have maximum positive impact for various socioeconomic, cultural, and ethnic groups.

Another area that deserves further exploration is the relationship of weight and health in the view of target population members. This study suggests that a heavier body weight is perceived as healthier, at least for some people and under certain conditions, and that this judgment may be related to an individual's ethnicity (Thompson and Story 2003: 35).

Conclusion

There you have it. The facts are the facts. African Americans and all Americans are becoming more overweight and obese than ever before. There is no doubt that this is an epidemic that appears to be out of control. With so much influence from the media, the fast-food industry, peer pressure, and family cultural patterns of eating, it is no wonder that our health status and quality of life are being adversely affected.

America has become a *culture of obesity*. Culture refers to the shared patterns and learned life ways particular to and representative of a group. Culture also means a system of shared beliefs, values, and traditions that are transmitted from generation to generation through learning. Besides the putative culture-bound phenomenon of excessive body fat, obese persons encounter other unique experiences not understood by persons of normal weight. In understanding the *culture of obesity*, one must also remember that there are notable variations between obese groups of differing gender, age, and ethnicity (Base-Smith and Campinha-Bacote 2003: 52).

We need to face this dilemma head on. Do we continue with the same pattern of unhealthy eating and misperception of exercise for the next decade or attempt to re-examine our eating patterns and revisit what it means to truly exercise in order to stop this epidemic in its tracks?

I strongly believe that we can stop this epidemic right in its tracks by re-examining our eating patterns, revisiting our exercise regimens, re-evaluating our perceptions of healthy and what we consider overweight and/or obese, and particularly reassessing our definitions of healthy and fit body image. Although this is a major task for all of us, it can be accomplished.

Of course, this first step begins and ends with you and me! That's why this book focuses on you, as an individual and an African American, to take an unbiased, serious and cultural look at your lifestyle and the negative effects it may have on your health and fitness. So let's continue on this journey together and find out what other African Americans believe about overweight, obesity, body image, exercise, and what it means to be healthy and fit—from an *African American perspective*!

Postevaluation Questions

1. How do the current statistics of overweight and obesity relate to the average African American?

 The current statistics on overweight and obesity relate to the average African American because the data reflects that the African American population on the average is getting much heavier than in previous years. This heavier weight, on average, results in increased chances of hypertension, diabetes, and heart disease.

2. How can health professionals encourage African Americans to recognize the significance of these overweight and obesity statistics?

 Health professionals can encourage African Americans to recognize the significance of overweight and obesity issues by talking about whether they want a better quality of life each and every day. The second step is to encourage African Americans to try to lose just a few pounds. If they do want to try to lose a few pounds, then the third step is for the health professional to suggest that by losing weight gradually, they will experience a better quality of life (more mobile, fewer aches and pains, and better breathing).

3.   How can African Americans begin to change these overweight and obesity statistics?

African Americans can change the overweight statistics by focusing on individual achievements in weight loss as well as to encourage others within their network of friends and family members to gradually modify and change habits to a more health-conscious behavior and lifestyle.

References

Allison, D., Fontaine, K., Manson, J., Stevens, J., and Van Itallie, T. 1999. Annual deaths attributable to obesity in the United States. *Journal of the American Medical Association* 282:1530–1538.

Base-Smith, V., and Campinha-Bacote, J. 2003. The culture of obesity. *Journal of National Black Nurses Association* 14(1):52–56.

Burke, G., Savage, P., and Manoko, T. 1992. Correlates of obesity in young black and white women: The CARDIA study. *American Journal of Public Health* 82:1621–1625.

Burton, B., Foster, W., Hirsch, J., and Van Itallie, T. 1985. Health implications of obesity: NIH consensus development conference. *International Journal of Obesity & Related Metabolic Disorders* 9:155–169.

CBS2-New York. 2005. Bill Clinton joins child obesity fight. Available at http:cbsnewyork.com/healthwatch/health_story_123150452.html.

Centers for Disease Control and Prevention. National Center for Health Statistics. 2004. Health behaviors of adults: United States, 1999–2001. Vital and Health Statistics. Series 10, Number 219. U.S. Department of Health and Human Services.

Centers for Disease Control and Prevention. The National Center for Health Statistics. 2002. Obesity still on the rise, new data show. Available at http://www.cdc.gov/nchs/releases/02news/obesityonrise.htm.

Centers for Disease Control and Prevention. The National Center for Chronic Disease Prevention and Health Promotion. 2002. Basics about overweight and obesity. Available at http://www.cdc.gov/nccdphp/dnpa/obesity/basics.htm.

Centers for Disease Control and Prevention. The National Center for Health Statistics. 1999. Prevalence of overweight and obesity among adults: United States, 1999–2002. Available at http://www.cdc.gov/nchs/products/pubs/pubd/hestats/obese/obse99.htm.

Clinton Foundation Organization. 2005. Press Release: Clinton Foundation and American Heart Association form alliance to create a healthier generation. Available at http:www.clintonfoundation.org/ 050305-nr-cf-hs-pr-wjc-and-american-heart-association-healthier-generation-initiative.htm.

Daniels, S., Arnett, D., Eckel, R., Gidding, S., Hayman, L., Kumanyika, S., Robinson, T., Scott, B., Jeor, S., and Williams, C. 2005. Overweight in children and adolescents: Pathophysiology, consequences, prevention, and treatment. *Circulation* 111:1999–2012.

Flegal, K., Carrol, M., Ogden, C., and Johnson, C. 2002. Prevalence and trends in obesity among U.S. adults, 1999–2000. *Journal of the American Medical Association* 288:1723–1727.

Flores, G., Fuentes-Afflick, E., Barbot, O., Carter-Pokras, O., Claudio, L., Lara, M., McLaurin, J., Pachter, L., Gomez, F., Mendoza, F., Valdez, R., Villarruel, A., Zambrana, R., Greenberg, R., and Weitzman, M. 2002. The health of Latino children: Urgent priorities, unanswered questions, and a research agenda. *Journal of the American Medical Association* 288:82–90.

Fontanarosa, P. 2002. Obesity research: A call for papers. *Journal of the American Medical Association* 288:1772–1773.

Garnett, C. 2002. Panel weighs in on diet, fat & cholesterol. *The NIH Record* 54:1, 8–9.

Gillum, R. 1987. Overweight and obesity in black women: A review of published data from the National Center for Health Statistics. *Journal of the National Medical Association* 79:865–871.

Gordon-Larsen, P., Adair, L., and Popkin, B. 2003. The relationship of ethnicity, socioeconomic factors, and overweight in U.S. adolescents. *Obesity Research* 11(1):121–129.

McTigue, K., Garrett., J., and Popkin, B. 2002. The natural history of the development of obesity in a cohort of young U.S. adults between 1981 and 1998. *Annals of Internal Medicine* 136:857–864.

Mokdad, A., Serdula, M., Dietz, W., Bowman, B., Marks, J., and Koplan, J. 1999. The spread of the obesity epidemic in the United States, 1991–1998. *Journal of the American Medical Association* 282:1519–1522.

Must, A., Spadano, J., Coakley, E., Field, A., Colditz, G., and Dietz, W. 1999. The disease burden associated with overweight and obesity. *Journal of the American Medical Association* 282:1523–1529.

National Center for Health Statistics. 1997. *Health United States 1996–97 and Injury Chartbook.* Hyattsville, MD: DHHS Publication PHS 97-1232.

National Heart, Lung and Blood Institute (NHLBI). National Institutes of Health. 1998. *Clinical Guidelines on the Identification, Evaluation, and Treatment of Overweight and Obesity in Adults: Executive Summary.* Hyattsville, MD: DHHS Publication PHS 98-4083.

Ogden, C., Flegal, K., Carroll, M., and Johnson, C. 2002. Prevalence and trends in overweight among U.S. children and adolescents, 1999–2000. *Journal of the American Medical Association* 288:1728–1732.

Olshansky, S., Passaro, D., Hershow, R., Layden, J., Carnes, B., Brody, J., Hayflick, L., Butler, R., Allison, D., and Ludwig, D. 2005. A potential decline in life expectancy in the United States in the 21st century. *New England Journal of Medicine* 352(11):1138–1145.

Peeke, P., Sacks, F., and Foster, G. 2002. Promoting healthy lives: Diet, fat & cholesterol. The NIH Record. 54(14):1, 8–9. U.S. Department of Health and Human Services.

Professional Guide to Diseases. 1998. Springhouse Corporation. Springhouse, PA: Springhouse Corporation.

Satcher, D. 2001. Overweight and obesity threatens U.S. health gains. U.S. Department of Health and Human Services Press Release, Thursday,

December 31, 2001. Available at http://www.surgeongeneral.gov/news/pressreleases/pr_obesity.htm.

Shavers, V., and Shankar, S. 2002. Trend in the prevalence of overweight and obesity among urban African American hospital employees and public housing residents. *Journal of the National Medical Association* 94:566–576.

Strauss, R., and Pollack, H. 2001. Epidemic increase in childhood overweight, 1986–1998. *Journal of the American Medical Association* 286:2845–2848.

Thompson, L., and Story, M. 2003. Perceptions of overweight and obesity in their community: Findings from focus groups with urban, African American caretakers of preschool children. *Journal of the National Black Nurses Association* 14:28–37.

Troiano, R., and Flegal, K. 1998. Overweight children and adolescents: Description, epidemiology, and demographics. *Pediatrics* 101(3):497–504.

Troiano, R., Flegal, K., Kuczmarski, R., Campbell, S., and Johnson, C. 1995. Overweight prevalence and trends for children and adolescents: The national health and nutrition examination surveys, 1963 to 1991. *Archives of Pediatric Adolescent Medicine* 149:1085–1091.

U.S. Department of Health & Human Services. 1997. *Health. United States 1996–97 and Injury Chartbook.* National Center for Health Statistics. Washington, DC: U.S. Government Printing Office. DHHS Publication No. 97–1232.

PART II
SOCIOCULTURAL ISSUES

This section presents four major issues that are not often addressed when investigating or developing weight-loss programs for the diverse African American population. They are Body Image Preferences, Food Preferences, Exercise and Physical Fitness Preferences, and Adding African American Culture to Health, Fitness, Diet, and Food Programs.

Body Image Preferences among African Americans

Critical Thinking Questions

1.   Do African Americans prefer a particular body type?
2.   What are the preferences of body images among African Americans?
3.   How do African Americans perceive a healthy body type?
4.   How do African Americans perceive an overweight and/or obese body type?

Introduction

I definitely realize that my book's topics on health, fitness, body image, and overweight touch on a number of sensitive issues within the African American community. In fact, most of these topics are so sensitive within the African American community that most African Americans are hesitant to talk about them for fear of being outcast by betraying this "black cultural code of silence" when issues hit too close to home. Let me tell you up front, I would be the first one to say, "Hey don't go there, you are talkin' about some issues that we hold dearly and closely to our soul so you better know what you're talkin' about and you better respect it!"

Indeed, I do understand the breadth of this sensitive cultural topic, and that is why I have done my homework and will present to you in a respectful manner my views and, of course, the views from the general African American community on body image, overweight, obesity, and good health. I believe that this has to be the starting point before any discussion how to address and solve the epidemic of overweight and obesity in our African American community that is affecting the young, the middle-aged, the elderly, the poor, the working poor, the middle class, the upper class, the men, and particularly the women—all of us!

Our Views on Body Image

How many times have you heard or used the following phrases?

"That boy needs some meat on his bones!"

"There is nothing wrong with him, he is just very healthy."

"I like my women thick with some hips on them."

"Why are you exercising, you are going to be too thin!"

"There is just more of me to love."

"There must be somethin' wrong with him/her because he/she looks like he/she lost some weight!"

These comments, and so many more, reflect the African American perspective that if one is to be healthy, he or she must be at least well-proportioned (noticeable hips, stomach, thighs, breasts) bordering on overweight and definitely not too thin (perceived indication of contracting HIV/AIDS or eating disorder such as bulimia/anorexia). Moreover, these comments reflect African Americans' "flexible cultural definition of healthiness." In other words, in the African American community, it is good to have some "meat on your bones" primarily because this body type indicates that the person is getting more than enough food to eat and that they have enough income and leisure time to consume these food products.

On one hand, this "flexible cultural definition of healthiness" is actually to the advantage of African Americans because it allows for varying degrees of acceptable body types within the culture, thereby preventing a narrow definition of which body type constitutes healthy. On the other hand, this "flexible cultural definition of healthiness" actually promotes the acceptance of overweight and obesity as the norm within the African American community. Therefore, the more accepted and ideal body type becomes the heavier person as opposed to the thinner one. Obviously, there are tremendous health and quality-of-life issues to take into account when the majority of the African American population adheres to this "flexible cultural definition of healthiness."

Nonetheless, African Americans' "flexible cultural definition of healthiness" is actually a definition that mainstream society wishes that it could truly embrace and make a part of its culture value pattern. Yet the preference for thinness within mainstream U.S. society has contributed to eating disorders such as anorexia and bulimia among white males and females. In addition to the cultural pattern of thinness, U.S. mainstream society receives constant messages and pressure from the media, the entertainment industry, the workplace, and the fitness industry to stay or to become thin.

So what is the mainstream definition of obesity and overweight and how does this definition compare with African Americans' perceptions of an obese or overweight body type? Moreover, what is the ideal body form (type) among African American men and women? In the next section, let's read how U.S. mainstream society, institutions, and experts define overweight and obesity.

Re-examining Criteria for Overweight, Obesity, and Body Mass Index in the United States

Overweight

The National Center for Chronic Disease Prevention and Health Promotion at the Centers for Disease Control and Prevention defines overweight as an increased body weight in relation to height, when compared with some standard of acceptable or desirable weight (Centers for Disease Control and Prevention 2003). This standard of acceptable or desirable weight is derived in three major ways:

- By using a mathematical formula known as body mass index (BMI), which represents weight levels associated with the lowest overall risk to health. Desirable BMI levels may vary with age.

- By using actual heights and weights measured and collected on people who are representative of the U.S. population by the National Center for Health Statistics.

- Other desirable weight tables have been created by the Metropolitan Life Insurance Company, based on their client populations.

The key issues regarding this U.S. definition of overweight are that it is based upon "a standard of acceptable or desirable weight"; it is calculated by the BMI; and it depends upon a representative sample of the U.S. population.

Interestingly, each of these key issues related to the U.S. definition of overweight conflict with the African American population. Why? It is very simple.

First, the U.S. definition of overweight is based on "a standard of acceptable or desirable weight" in accordance with mainstream society's values and standards but not in accordance with the majority of the African American population. Mainstream society tends to have a standard or desirable weight that follows a "thin" concept versus the African American standard for desirable weight that follows a "fuller and/or well-rounded" concept of desirable weight. Thus, this U.S. definition of overweight already conflicts with the African American perspective of what constitutes overweight.

Second, overweight is calculated by the BMI. Although the BMI is used regularly in clinical and research assessment, the BMI has been challenged regularly by numerous researchers and their research publications as to its accurate measurement as a predictor of chronic disease development among various overweight populations.

Third, the U.S. definition of overweight depends on a representative sample of U.S. citizens including African Americans. Unfortunately, in most national medical and health-care studies of Americans, the African American population has been poorly represented. The major issues concerning the African American population in national studies involve not only the lower number of African Americans in national studies but also the obtaining of a diverse sample of African Americans living in urban, rural, and suburban areas across this country. If these two issues are not accounted for in national studies, then there is a degree of uncertainty as to the accuracy of national samples that claim to reflect the African American population.

Obesity

Obesity is defined as an excessively high amount of body fat or adipose tissue in relation to lean body mass (Centers for Disease Control and Prevention 2003). The amount of body fat (or adiposity) includes concern for both the distribution of fat throughout the body and the size of adipose tissue deposits.

Body Mass Index

Body mass index is a common measure expressing the relationship (or ratio) of weight to height. It is a mathematical formula in which a person's body weight in kilograms is divided by the square of his or her height in meters (i.e., kg/m^2). The BMI is more highly correlated with body fat than any other indicator of height and weight (Centers for

Disease Control and Prevention 2003). Individuals with a BMI of 25 to 29.9 are considered overweight, and individuals with a BMI of 30 or more are considered obese.

Well, I wanted to see how this BMI applies to my current weight situation so I took the test at the National Heart, Lung, and Blood Institute (NIH) Web site (www.nhlbisupport.com/bmi/). The instructions are as follows:

1. Enter your weight and height using English or metric measures.
2. Click on compute and your BMI will appear in the heart of the figure.
3. See "Assessing Your Risk" for the health risks associated with overweight and obesity.

I entered 157 for my weight and 5' 4" for my height. I clicked the compute BMI button and it calculated my BMI score to be 27.0. According to the BMI categories, the score 27.0 falls in the middle of the overweight category (25.0–29.9). I am therefore overweight!

Of course, I wholeheartedly disagree! As an ex-athlete who follows a healthy exercise and diet regimen, I was astonished that my BMI score placed me into the overweight category. I then wondered, do I get punished for working out regularly and having a body type or form that is similar to other professional athletes or body builders and not typical of the average American? I think I do and I think there are others (African Americans) whose body form or type does not fit into the BMI categories and who, unfortunately, get categorized into a heavier BMI category.

Let it be known that I am not disputing the predictability factor of the BMI for increased mortality. The BMI can be used by the general public to assess a person's risk for chronic disease and illness, because the BMI is easily calculated and is therefore accessible to the general public (Fernandez et al. 2003). I am, however, disputing the very rigid and strict categories of the BMI as it relates to populations that may have a different body build and form than the statistically measured and sampled mainstream American population.

Researchers are finally challenging the rigidness of the BMI. For example, Wagner and Heyward (2000) emphasize the following from their study entitled "Measures of Body Composition in Blacks and Whites: A Comparative Review:"

> *"We believe that more research is needed regarding the influence of race on BMI because this could have implications for the false assessment of the prevalence of obesity."*

"We urge body-composition researchers to collect and report socioeconomic, ethnic, and environmental background data in future studies. This information, combined with the emerging advances in genetic research, could lead to a better understanding of the differences in body composition between racial or ethnic groups and the prevalence of obesity-related diseases." (Wagner and Heward 2000: 1400)

For example, in the *American Journal of Clinical Nutrition* article entitled "Is Percentage Body Fat Differentially Related to Body Mass Index in Hispanic Americans, African Americans, and European Americans," the researchers investigated whether the relation between percentage body fat (PBF) and body mass index (BMI) in adult Hispanic Americans (HAs) differed from that of African Americans (AAs) and European Americans (EAs). From a sample of 487 men and 933 women, the researchers found that for men, their results showed no significant differences between Hispanic Americans and European Americans, African Americans and European Americans, and Hispanic Americans and African Americans.

Among their sample of women, however, their results showed that the relation between PBF and BMI in Hispanic American women differs from that of European American and African American women. Specifically, at BMI less than 30, Hispanic American women tended to have higher PBF than did European American and African American women. For BMI greater than 35, European American women tended to have higher PBF than did Hispanic American and African American women (Fernandez et al. 2003).

In general, this study was one of the first to investigate whether the relation between PBF and BMI in Hispanic Americans differs from that in African Americans and European Americans. The findings showed that at the same BMI, women of Hispanic American ethnicity have different PBF values when compared with women of European American and African American descent. Although there are some potential explanations for these differences, including sedentary lifestyles and possible differences in genetic makeup among the ethnic groups, the mechanisms underlying these differences require further investigation.

Research Studies on African Americans' Body Image and Body Type Preferences

In order to better understand African Americans' body image and body type preferences, let's begin with a baseline definition of the issues. According to psychologists, *body image* is the internal, subjective representation of physical appearance and bodily experience, whereas *body type* preference is the ideal against which one measures or compares one's own body's size and shape (Thompson and Smolak 2001). In other words, body image is your perception of how your body looks, and body type is how your body compares with other body types. These two concepts—body image and body type preference—are very important factors as to why African Americans have this (what I refer to as) "flexible cultural definition of healthiness."

In this section, I am going to highlight several recent studies that examined body image, body size, and body type preferences in the African American population and other U.S. populations. This section is subdivided into four age-based and school-based groupings: (1) Elementary, (2) Middle School and High School, (3) College, and (4) Professional Adults. The grouping of African Americans into specific age-based and school-based categories will provide you with a better understanding of the variation and diversity of opinions within the African American population with regard to body image, body size, and body type preferences.

Elementary

To examine the prevalence of overweight concerns and body dissatisfaction among third-grade girls and boys and the influences of ethnicity and socioeconomic status (SES), I present a study conducted in thirteen northern California public elementary schools, entitled "Overweight Concerns and Body Dissatisfaction among Third-Grade Children: The Impacts of Ethnicity and Socioeconomic Status." This research study assessed overweight concerns, body dissatisfaction, and desired shape, height, and weight among 969 children (mean age, 8.5 years) (Robinson et al. 2001).

Of the 999 third-grade children enrolled in the thirteen schools, 969 (97.0%) participated in the study. Parents refused participation for 29 children, and 1 child was absent during the study. The sample consisted of 44 percent white, 21 percent Latino, 19 percent Asian American (not including Filipino), 8 percent Filipino, 5 percent African American, 1 percent American Indian, and 1 percent Pacific Islander. Slightly over 50 percent (50.2%) were girls, and boys were slightly older (8.5 years vs. 8.4 years) than girls in the sample. The responses from the Kids' Eating Disorders Survey (KEDS) provided the data for the research team (Robinson et al. 2001).

As hypothesized, the researchers found that girls reported greater overweight concerns, greater body dissatisfaction, and thinner desired body shapes than boys. After sex differences were found, ethnic differences were assessed separately for boys and girls. Among girls, African Americans had significantly more overweight concerns than Asian Americans and Filipinos, and Latinas had significantly more overweight concerns than whites, Asian Americans, and Filipinas. White and Latina girls reported greater body dissatisfaction than Asian American girls (Robinson et al. 2001: 184).

To examine whether ethnic differences could be explained by differences in actual body fatness, comparisons were repeated after stratifying girls into three BMI groups: girls with a BMI $\leq$ 25th percentile for the entire sample, girls with a BMI between 25th and 75th percentiles, and girls with a BMI $\geq$ 75th percentile. Data indicated that overweight concerns and body dissatisfaction increased with increasing BMI in all ethnic groups. After groups were stratified by BMI, significant ethnic differences in overweight concerns persisted only in the large middle stratum. Among these girls, Latinas reported significantly more overweight concerns than whites and Asian Americans, and there was a trend toward greater overweight concerns among African Americans compared with whites (p = .05). There were no significant differences in body dissatisfaction or desired body shape among girls or among boys (Robinson et al. 2001: 184).

Overall, this study indicates that African American and Hispanic girls are not immune to cultural emphasis on extreme thinness. Latina and African American third-grade girls reported greater or equivalent levels of dysfunctional eating attitudes and behaviors in comparison with white girls, even after controlling for actual body fatness and SES. The findings suggest that body dissatisfaction and overweight concerns are prevalent across sex, ethnicity, and socioeconomic class. It also indicates a need for culturally appropriate school-based primary prevention programs designed specifically for Latino and African American children (Robinson et al. 2001: 186).

To determine if body image, size, or preferences are formulated earlier than junior high or high school years, I present a study entitled "Ideal Body Size Beliefs and Weight Concerns of Fourth-Grade Children." This research study assessed racial and gender differences in perceptions of ideal body size among white and black fourth-grade children (Thompson, Corwin, and Sargent 1997).

The researchers surveyed a random sample of fourth-graders at small, medium, and large South Carolina elementary schools. The final sample of participants consisted of 817 white (51.8%), African American (48.2%), female (51.4%), and male (48.6%) fourth-graders aged 8 to 12 years (mean age = 9.3 years). The survey collected information in the following areas: dieting and weight concern, body image and body size perception, and demographics.

When students were asked to select a picture that "looks most like you," the researchers found that among these fourth-graders, African American males selected a larger self than white males. Additionally, African American females selected a significantly heavier size for self than white females. As for selecting an ideal female and male child size,

African American females selected a larger female child size as ideal than white females (Thompson, Corwin, and Sargent 1997: 283).

Overall, this study indicates that even at this point in the sociocultural development of children, the factors of gender, socioeconomic status, and ethnicity are of great influence in selecting ideal body size and determining body size satisfaction. African American children selected significantly *heavier ideal sizes* than white children for self, male child, adult male, and adult female (Thompson, Corwin, and Sargent 1997: 284).

Similarly, in the study entitled "Discrepancies in Body Image Perception among Fourth-Grade Public School Children from Urban, Suburban, and Rural Maryland," researchers found that African American elementary children chose larger figures than did whites and other races to represent their current and ideal images and were most satisfied with their body size. The objective of this study was to determine whether there is an association between body image perception and weight status as measured by the body mass index among a group of fourth-graders in Maryland (Welch et al. 2004).

The sample consisted of 524 fourth-grade public school students (54% girls, 46% boys) from three geographically distinct regions in Maryland (38.6% urban, 30.7% suburban, 30.7% rural). Of the total sample of 524 students, 60.7 percent (318) were white, 30.9 percent (162) African American, 3.4 percent (18) Hispanic, 2.1 percent (11) Asian/Pacific Islander, and 2.9 percent (15) Other. Approximately 39 percent of the students were from an urban setting, and the other two geographic locations were equally represented (surburban 30.7%, rural 30.7%) (Welch et al. 2004: 1081).

The researchers used silhouettes of children (referred to as Collins figures) to test their sample's body image perception. The pictorials consisted of images of girls and boys, numbered 1 to 7, to correspond with increases in size from very thin to obese. Fourth-graders were asked to select images that most looked like them (current body image) and that looked the way they wanted to look (ideal body image). A body image discrepancy score was calculated by subtracting ideal body image from current body image. These scores were then sorted into three categories: (a) desires to be thinner (discrepancy scores greater than zero), (b) satisfied with current image (discrepancy scores equal to zero), and (c) desires to be bigger (discrepancy scores less than zero).

The researchers found that current body image scores did not differ significantly for boys and girls. However, boys had a significantly larger ideal image than girls. Approximately 47 percent of the fourth-graders were satisfied with their current image; the others either wanted to be smaller (42%) or larger (11%). Urban children had a higher ideal image than their suburban and rural counterparts. Additionally, more children from rural areas (47.2%) than urban areas (38.6%) wanted to lose weight (Welch et al. 2004: 1082).

Most importantly, the study's results found that African American students had a significantly higher current image and higher ideal image score than white students and other race/ethnicity students. In other words, African American fourth-graders selected significantly larger figures to represent their current and ideal images than did white, Hispanic, Asian/Pacific Islander, and other students (Welch et al. 2004: 1084).

Overall, the research team suggests that the results of their study highlight the fact that body image preferences begin early in life; therefore, caregivers, educators, and health professionals need to be mindful of the messages they send young children. Dietitians, in particular, using culturally appropriate materials, can educate students and adults about healthy weight, nutrition, exercise, and body image (Welch et al. 2004: 1084).

Middle School and High School

In another highlighted study, entitled "Body Image and Weight Concerns among African American and White Adolescent Females; Differences that Make a Difference," the researchers examined body image and dieting behaviors among African American and white adolescent females (Parker et al. 1995). They explored specifically the cultural factors that have an impact on weight perception, body image, beauty, and style.

In this study, 250 girls were recruited while they were in the eighth grade (junior high) and ninth grade (senior high school). Informants were 75 percent white, 16 percent Mexican American, and 9 percent Asian Americans. In the final year of the project, a second sample of 46 African American adolescent girls, drawn from grades 9–12 and other community groups in the same city, was added to the study. Their study of African American adolescent girls utilized both ethnographic interview and survey methods. Ten focus group discussions with four to five girls per group were conducted by African American researchers in order to identify the perceptions and concerns that African American girls held about their weight, body image, dieting, and other broader health and lifestyle factors (Parker et al. 1995: 105).

The research team consisted of both white and African American researchers. Focus group and individual interviews were transcribed, read, and discussed by members of the research team. Cultural differences and similarities that emerged from the data were analyzed in weekly meetings among the researchers. Later, a panel of community members were asked to comment on findings (Parker et al. 1995: 105).

The researchers stated that what was particularly striking in African American girls' descriptions, when compared with those of white adolescents, was the de-emphasis on external beauty as a prerequisite for popularity. As one girl noted,

> *"There's a difference between being just fine or being just pretty... because I know a lot of girls who aren't just drop-dead fine but they are pretty, and they're funny, all those things come in and that makes the person beautiful. There are a lot of bad-looking (physically beautiful) girls out there, but you can't stand being around them."* (Parker et al. 1995: 108)

The researchers also stated that girls were aware that African American boys had more specific physical criteria for an "ideal girl" than they had themselves. They commented that boys like girls who are shapely, "thick," and who had "nice thighs." One girl noted that

> *"guys would be talkin' about the butt... it be big."* (Parker et al. 1995: 108)

Another girl explained:

> *"I think pretty matters more to guys than to me. I don't care. Just real easy to talk to, that would be the ideal girl for me, but the ideal girl from the guy's perspective would be entirely different. They want them to be fine, you know what guys like, shapely. Black guys like black girls who are thick—full figured."* (Parker et al. 1995: 108)

Additionally, in focus group interviews, the researchers asked girls if they heard or engaged in much talk about being fat with their friends:

> *"I don't hear that a lot. I hang out with black people and they don't care—we don't worry if we're fat because we'd all be drawn away from that. We want to talk about what's going on, you know, about where we're going for lunch. We're not concerned with that."* (Parker et al. 1995: 108)

As for the issue of beauty, the researchers found that beauty was not described in relation to a particular size or set of body statistics. Girls noted that beauty was not merely a question of shape. It was more to be beautiful on the inside as well as on the outside, and to be beautiful a girl had to "know her culture." One girl explained that

> *"African American girls have inner beauty in themselves that they carry with them—their sense of pride."* (Parker et al. 1995: 108)

This sense of pride was commonly described as a legacy they received from their mothers (Parker et al. 1995: 108).

Overall, the researchers stated that from their study, the standards for body image and beauty among these African American adolescents can be summed up in what these girls term "looking good." "Looking good" or "got it goin' on" entails making what you've got work for you by creating and presenting a sense of style (Parker et al. 1995: 108).

College

Another study that I want to highlight is Altabe's (1998) study, entitled "Ethnicity and Body Image: Quantitative and Qualitative Analysis." Altabe (1998) conducted a survey among 150 males and 185 females who were college students attending the University of South Florida. Participants completed four different body image questionnaires as well as several self-ratings relating to appearance including (1) physical attractiveness and (2) physical appearance on a scale from 1 to 11 (Altabe 1998: 155).

Qualitative results from the sampled African Americans, Asian Americans, Caucasian Americans, and Hispanic Americans revealed that height was valued by all groups. All the female groups and the Asian and Caucasian males wanted to be thinner. All the males and the African American and Caucasian females wanted to be more toned. Non-Caucasian females wanted longer hair. All groups valued dark or wanted darker skin except for African American females and Asian males (Altabe 1998: 157).

For general appearance body image, African Americans had the most positive self-view, whereas Caucasians and Hispanics showed distinct differences. Asian Americans placed the least importance on physical appearance. Thus ethnic differences occurred for both weight and non-weight dimensions of body image (Altabe 1998: 158).

Another college-age based study that I want to highlight is a research study entitled "Comparisons of Body Image Dimensions by Race/Ethnicity and Gender in a University Population." The research team's major objectives were (1) to examine gender and race/ethnicity and the interaction of the two on body image dimensions; (2) to include three racial/ethnic groups; (3) to more comprehensively measure body image by assessing feelings about body parts significant to race/ethnicity; (4) to measure and control for numerous important possible confounds including age, body size, SES, and social desirability (Miller et al. 2000).

Participants were 120 college students from a northeastern (n = 27) and southwestern (n = 93) university. There were 20 male and 20 female students in each of three racial/ethnic groups: African American, European American, and Latino Americans. At the northeastern university, students were recruited from fourteen graduate or undergraduate classes in nine departments with the permission of the instructors. At the southwestern university, participants were solicited through the research pool (primarily undergraduates) of the Department of Psychology and given class credit for their participation (Miller et al. 2000: 312).

The researchers found that African Americans scored significantly higher than European Americans and Latino Americans on Appearance Evaluation and Body Areas Satisfaction and above European Americans on the Body Esteem Scale (BES). On the other appearance dimensions, African American women rated themselves significantly higher on Sexual Attractiveness than did European American women, with Latinas scoring in the middle. African American women also scored higher than other women on BES Weight Concern, showing a higher sense of self-esteem regarding their weight. Male groups did not differ on the BES (Miller et al. 2000: 314–315).

Overall, the research team suggests that their study helps to expand the database on differences and similarities in body image based on gender and race/ethnicity. It gives evidence of the need to expand the variables under consideration and to place them within the cultural context in an understanding of identity, self-esteem, and self-care (Miller et al. 2000: 315).

Professional Adults

A study entitled "Does Ethnicity Influence Body-Size Preference? A Comparison of Body Image and Body Size" examined body image and body-size assessments in a large sample of men and women of four ethnicities/races: black, Hispanic, Asian, and white. The researchers hypothesized that black women and men would report less body dissatisfaction than the other ethnic groups; black and Hispanic men and women, compared with Asians and whites, would accept heavier female figures and would select larger sizes as representing overweight and obese female figures (i.e., would have higher thresholds for what they consider obesity); regardless of ethnicity, women would be more dissatisfied with their size and shape than men; and women, compared with men, would select thinner female figures as attractive and acceptable (Cachelin et al. 2002: 160).

From this study of 1,229 participants (801 women and 428 men) of which 288 were Asian, 548 Hispanic, 208 African American, and 185 white, the researchers found that Asian women chose a somewhat larger female figure as being underweight than did African American women; and Asian women reported less body dissatisfaction than the other groups. In terms of the interaction between gender and race, white women chose the thinnest and African American men the heaviest female figure as attractive to men (Cachelin et al. 2002).

In summary, this study investigated body image and perceptions of attractive, acceptable, and typical female figures, across a range of sizes from underweight to obese, in a large community sample of Asian, African American, Hispanic, and white men and women. Wide ranges of age, educational level, and BMI were represented, and differences among groups of these variables were controlled. The findings suggested that ethnicity alone does not markedly influence perceptions of female body size. However, cultural acceptance of larger sizes may produce the tendency to be overweight in the first place (Cachelin et al. 2002: 165). This cultural acceptance of larger sizes directly applies to the African American community.

Another study that I am presenting is entitled "Body Image Preferences among Urban African Americans and Whites from Low Income Communities." The purpose of this study was to determine: (1) how African American and white men and women from similar low-income communities perceive their body mass relative to others in the population; and (2) whether ethnic and gender differences exist in the selection of ideal body image sizes for the same and opposite sex. Overall, the researchers designed this study as a community study to determine ethnic differences in the relative accuracy of self-estimates of body size (body image) and preferences for ideal body image in African American and white low-income communities (Becker et al. 1999).

This study was conducted in East Baltimore where adjacent urban African American and white communities of similar low socioeconomic status reside. Nine hundred twenty-seven persons were interviewed during eight weeks and asked to provide their height and weight and to select body size images from a standardized ethnic-specific Figure Rating Scale to represent their current self, ideal self, and their estimation of ideals for the opposite sex. The sample consisted of 579 African Americans (47% male, 53% female) and 348 whites (46% male, 54% female).

The researchers found that average ideal body image size for self was the same for African American men and white men, while African American women had a significantly greater ideal image size compared with white women. Interestingly, the ideal body image for white women was most distant from the image selected for their current self. Slightly more than one-fourth of white women were satisfied with their current body image, whereas more than one-half of African American women were satisfied with their current image (Becker et al. 1999: 381).

Additionally, the researchers found that African American men indicated a preference for *larger* body images in African American women than did white men for white women. African American women preferred a slightly larger body image for African American men compared with their white counterparts.

In general, the researchers state that their findings support earlier studies in special populations suggesting that a social norm may exist on a community-wide level that enables the acceptance of larger body images in African American women (Pulvers et al. 2004). Furthermore, this study suggests that there are ethnic differences in body image concepts that necessitate developing unique healthy weight strategies within lower socioeconomic communities. Relative to overweight, the apparently different perceptions of African Americans and whites call for health strategies that address cultural and not just socioecomic status (Becker et al. 1999).

Conclusion

So what kind of conclusion have you derived from the information that I presented to you? In the last section of this chapter, I presented to you research studies across the United States in varying age- and school-based categories (elementary, middle and high school, college, and professional adults) examining the issues of body image and body preferences among African American adults, adolescents, and children and realizing that African Americans significantly select larger body types as the ideal and for self when compared with whites. In the beginning part of this chapter, I presented the basic definitions of overweight, obesity, and body mass index. I even challenged the use of the body mass index, particularly its usage among various ethnic populations (i.e., African Americans and Hispanic Americans). Finally, I began this chapter with the contention that African Americans have a "flexible cultural definition of healthiness" thereby allowing us to appreciate, admire, and emulate larger body types as the cultural norm for males and females.

The results of several studies indicate that African Americans have an ideal body type and preference of body image that are different from those of other groups (Brown and Konner 1987; Stevens, Kumanyika, and Keil 1994; Dounchis, J., Hayden, H., and Wilfley, D. 2001; Smolak, L., and Levine, M. 2001; Gore 1999; Pulvers et al. 2004). In fact, we need to keep in mind positive aspects of African American culture as it relates to body image, body type, and preferences. As Baskin, Ahluwalia, and Resnicow (2001) stated in their article, "Obesity Intervention among African American Children and Adolescents,"

> *"Thus, rather than holding whites and majority culture as the ideal, it may be important to incorporate the positive elements of black culture regarding body image and food rather than attempting to shift their values toward those of European Americans."* (Baskin, Ahluwalia, and Resnicow 2001: 1036)

I wholeheartedly agree with this statement and we as African Americans must continue to feel good about our appearance and base our body image within our own culture, thereby embracing more of ourselves (mentally and physically) and collectively as a people.

Postevaluation Questions

1. Should health professionals challenge the image of the preferred body type among African Americans?

   Health professionals should not initially challenge the image of the preferred body type among African Americans primarily because there are a wide array of cultural attachments to these body images. However, after a thorough discussion with the individual African American results in the conclusion that the individual African American would like a different body type, additional consultation should follow to find out specifically the body type most preferred.

2. Should health professionals challenge African American body images of what constitutes a "healthy" person versus an "overweight" person?

   As stated in question #1, health professionals should not initially challenge African American body images of what constitutes a healthy person versus an overweight person. Preferred body images among African Americans are often different from mainstream audiences. Therefore, the health professional should gradually inquire about the patient's definition of healthy versus overweight and then discuss the differences in health and medical consequences between the two body images.

3. How can African Americans change the perspectives of health professionals regarding their perception of what constitutes healthy and overweight for African Americans?

   African Americans should try to open up more of a dialogue with their health professionals regarding their beliefs, values, and attitudes associated with preferred body images, healthy body types, and overweight body types.

References

Altabe, M. 1998. Ethnicity and body image: Quantitative and qualitative analysis. *International Journal of Eating Disorders* 23:153–159.

Baskin, M., Ahluwalia, H., and Resnicow, K. 2001. Obesity intervention among African American children and adolescents. *Pediatric Clinics of North America* 48:1027–1039.

Becker, D., Yanek, L., Koffman, D., and Bronner, Y. 1999. Body image preferences among urban African Americans and whites from low income communities. *Ethnicity & Disease* 9:377–386.

Brown, P., and Konner, M. 1987. An anthropological perspective on obesity. *Annals of the New York Academy of Sciences* 499:29–46.

Cachelin, F., Rebeck, R., Chung, G., and Pelayo, E. 2002. Does ethnicity influence body-size preference? A comparison of body image and body size. *Obesity Research* 10:158–166.

Centers for Disease Control and Prevention. 2003. Overweight and obesity: Defining overweight and obesity. Available at http://www.cdc.gov/nccdphp/dnpa/obesity/definig.htm.

Dounchis, J., Hayden, H., and Wilfley, D. 2001. Obesity, body image and eating disorders in ethnically diverse children and adolescents. In K. Thompson and L. Smolak (Eds.), *Body Image, Eating Disorders and Obesity in Youth*. Washington, DC: American Psychological Association, 67–90.

Fernandez, J., Moonseon, H., Heymsfield, S., Pierson, R., Pi-Sunyer, F., Wang, Z., Wang, J., Hayes, M., Allison, D., and Gallgher, D. 2003. Is percentage body fat differentially related to body mass index in Hispanic Americans, African Americans, and European Americans? *American Journal of Clinical Nutrition* 77:71–75.

Gore, S. 1999. African American women's perceptions of weight: Paradigm shift for advanced practice. *Holistic Nursing Practice* 13:71–79.

Miller, K., Gleaves, D., Hirsch, T., Green, B., Snow, A., and Corbett, C. 2000. Comparisons of body image dimensions by race/ethnicity and gender in a university population. *International Journal of Eating Disorders* 27:310–316.

Parker, S., Nichter, M., Nichter, M., Vuckovic, S. C., and Ritenbaugh, C. 1995. Body image and weight concerns among African American and white adolescent females: Differences that make a difference. *Human Organization* 54:103–114.

Pulvers, K., Lee, R., Kaur, H., Mayo, M., Flitzgibbon, M., Jeffries, S., Butler, J., Hou, Q., and Ahluwalia, J. 2004. Development of a culturally relevant body image instrument among urban African Americans. *Obesity Research* 12(10):1641–1651.

Robinson, T., Chang, J., Haydel, K., and Killen, J. 2001. Overweight concerns and body dissatisfaction among third-grade children: The impacts of ethnicity and socioeconomic status. *Journal of Pediatrics* 138:181–187.

Smolak, L., and Levine, M. 2001. Body image in children. In K. Thompson and L. Smolak (Eds.), *Body Image, Eating Disorders and Obesity in Youth*. Washington, DC: American Psychological Association, 41–66.

Stevens, J., Kumanyika, S., and Keil, J. 1994. Attitudes toward body size and dieting: differences between elderly black and white women. *American Journal of Public Health* 84:1322–1325.

Thompson, K., and Smolak, L. (Eds.). 2001. *Body Image, Eating Disorders and Obesity in Youth.* Washington, DC: American Psychological Association.

Thompson, S., Corwin, S., and Sargent, R. 1997. Ideal body size beliefs and weight concerns of fourth-grade children. *International Journal of Eating Disorders* 21:279–284.

Wagner, D., and Heyward, V. 2000. Measures of body composition in blacks and whites: A comparative review. *American Journal of Clinical Nutrition* 71:1392–1402.

Welch, C., Gross, S., Bronner, Y., Dewberry-Moore, D., and Paige, D. 2004. Discrepancies in body image perception among fourth-grade public school children from urban, suburban, and rural Maryland. *Journal of the American Dietetic Association* 1040:1080–1085.

Food Preferences among African Americans

Critical Thinking Questions

1. Is there a distinguishable set of foods that African Americans prefer?
2. How did this set of food preferences become established in the African American community?
3. How is "soul food" viewed in the African American community?
4. Why do a large percentage of African Americans adhere to the traditional soul food pattern?

Introduction

When I was growing up, I often wondered why I preferred certain types of foods more than others and if my selections of these certain types of foods were a reflection of my individual food preferences, my family's food preferences, my ethnic group's food preferences, or society's food preferences? Now I can see that my preference for certain types of foods were and still are a reflection of all those factors and more.

The fact that my preference for certain foods that have been labeled as "soul food" reflects my connection to my African American heritage, my family's history, my regional history, and my individual history is quite similar to the experience of many other African Americans in the United States. Yet today, I am more aware of some of the unhealthy and healthy aspects of my current African American dietary pattern.

Recent Studies on the Dietary Pattern of African Americans

Because relatively little is still known of the dietary pattern among African Americans, a group of researchers conducted a re-examination of a select sample of African Americans in a diabetes-related study. In a report entitled "Fruit, Vegetable and Fat Intake in a Population-Based Sample of African Americans," Gary et al. (2004) conducted a cross-sectional analysis of 2,172 African American adults in Project DIRECT (Diabetes Interventions Reaching and Educating Communities Together) and a baseline assessment of a sample population from Raleigh and Greensboro, North Carolina, of their daily fruit, vegetable, and fat intake. They found that a very small number of participants met national recommendations for average servings of fruit and vegetables.

The study's sample of 2,172 African Americans was predominately female (62%) and had a mean age of 46 years. About 38 percent of participants were currently married, and the majority were employed (61%). Most participants had completed high school and about one-third had yearly incomes equal to or greater than $25,000.

Interestingly, most participants (81%) rated their overall health as being excellent, very good, or good. However, about two-thirds of participants were overweight or obese. About one-third reported that they were attempting to lose weight, and 21 percent had a doctor recommend that they lose weight (Gary et al. 2004: 1602).

Overall, the evaluation of fruit and vegetable intake stratified by health status showed no significant patterns. Only 8 percent of 2,172 Project DIRECT participants reported eating at least two servings of fruit per day, and only 3 percent reported eating three or more. Likewise only 16 percent reported eating at least three servings of vegetables per day, and 6 percent reported eating four or more. Overall, the dietary patterns of participants fell far below recommendations (Gary et al. 2004: 1602).

However participants who were overweight or obese, who were attempting weight loss, or who had a doctor recommend that they lose weight reported significantly more daily fruit and vegetable intake than participants who did not experience these concerns. Those who had been physically active in the past month had a significantly higher intake of fruits and vegetables than those who had not been physically active (Gary et al. 2004: 1602).

Moreover, older participants reported significantly less daily total and saturated fat intake than did younger participants. Although women reported a higher daily total fat intake than did men, they reported a significantly lower intake from saturated fat. Daily total fat and saturated fat intake were significantly lower in participants who had at least a college degree than in those with less than a high school education (Gary et al. 2004: 1602).

Although this study's results were comparable with other major studies (Neumark-Sztainer et al. 2002), the data had several limitations such as the fact that the data were self-reported and that no inferences could be made for causal associations. Nonetheless, this latest study of African American dietary pattern provides some supportive evidence that African Americans dietary pattern does not meet national standards with regard to recommended fruit and vegetable intake.

Another study that I want to highlight is entitled "Eating at Fast-Food Restaurants is Associated with Dietary Intake, Demographic, Psychosocial and Behavioral Factors among African Americans in North Carolina." The research team's major objectives were:

1.   To describe the prevalence of eating at fast-food restaurants among African American adults in North Carolina; and

2.   To examine cross-sectional associations of eating at fast-food restaurants with dietary intake and demographic, behavioral, and diet-related psychosocial factors in this population. (Satia, Galanko, and Siega-Riz 2004: 1090)

The study's results are based on a population-based cross-sectional survey of 658 African Americans, aged 20–70 years, in North Carolina. An eleven-page questionnaire assessed eating at fast-food restaurants, demographic, behavioral, and diet-related psychosocial factors, and dietary intake (fruit, vegetable, total fat and saturated fat intake, and fat-related dietary behaviors).

The demographics of the African American participants were as follows: 41 percent were male, 43.9 ± 11.6 years (mean), 37 percent were college graduates or had an advanced degree, more than half (56%) were married, 35 percent were overweight, 40 percent were obese, and 82 percent were from urban counties. Only 14 percent of respondents were current smokers, and 41 percent reported current multivitamin use (Satia, Galanko, and Siega-Riz 2004:1092).

The research team found the following results:

1.   Seventy-six percent reported eating at a fast-food restaurant during the previous three months.

2.   The frequency of eating at fast-food restaurants was positively and linearly associated with total fat and saturated fat intakes and fat-related dietary behaviors.

3.   Participants who reported usually/often eating at fast-food restaurants were more often younger, never married, and physically inactive.

4.   Frequency of eating at fast-food restaurants was positively associated with obesity (mean BMI 31.3).

5. Participants who usually/often eat at fast-food restaurants were also more likely to be dissatisfied with their weight and taking steps to lose weight.

6. Frequency of eating at fast-food restaurants was not associated with financial ability to purchase healthy foods, need for information on how to prepare healthy foods and meals, or knowledge of the Food Guide Pyramid. (Satia, Galanko, and Siega-Riz 2004: 1092)

Based on these findings, the researchers suggest that interventions to reduce consumption of fast foods should address attitudes about diet–disease relationships and convenience barriers to healthy eating (Schlundt, Hargreaves, and Buchowski 2003). More broadly, educational efforts to improve dietary intake and reduce obesity must consider both demographic and behavioral characteristics and address away-from-home eating, particularly at fast-food establishments (Sati, Glanko, and Siega-Riz 2004: 1095).

Food, Food Habits, and African Americans

According to *Webster's Dictionary*, *food* is defined as any substance that provides the nutrients necessary to maintain life and growth when ingested. When food is ingested and consumed in a regular pattern, we are referring to *food habits* (Kittler and Suchler 2000: 2).

Food habits refers to the ways in which humans use food, how food is obtained and stored, how it is prepared, how it is served and to whom, and how it is consumed (Kittler and Sucher 2000: 2; Fieldhouse 1992). For example, research by Airhihenbuwa et al. (1996) on African American eating patterns found that not only did the issues of *belongingness* and *status* play a part in eating patterns but also the *cultural attitudes* about where and with whom food is eaten emerged as being equivalent in importance to attitudes about specific foods. In the study entitled "Cultural Aspects of African American Eating Patterns," Airhihenbuwa et al. (1996) investigated the following key issues:

- Food habits that have been described consistently as characteristics in African American culture dating from slavery to determine whether these food practices were perceived as important cultural traditions

- Perceived need to preserve certain practices in spite of their association with health problems

- Whether certain potentially favorable food habits were being perpetuated for their perceived health benefits

- Psychosocial aspects of eating that could be important influences on the potential for food behavior change. (Airhihenbuwa et al. 1996: 246)

Using focus group interviews and then qualitative analyses to analyze the focus group data among the sample of African Americans (21 males and 32 females, aged 13–65 years from low- and middle-income urban communities in South Central Pennsylvania), Airhihenbuwa et al. (1996) highlighted three major themes:

1. Association of food choices with being black
2. Issues related to the context of eating
3. Healthfulness of soul food and other traditional food practices.

With regard to theme no. 1 (association of food choices with being black), participants were prompted to discuss how they thought that being black affected their food choices, whether this was different for older persons, and whether this was different for higher income blacks. One male youth said that he didn't care who made the food and another female youth stated:

"Black people will eat anything."

Yet for older participants, food choices of black Americans were distinctly influenced by custom as well as by slavery and discrimination. For example:

"Blacks eat what they are accustomed to eat."

"I think, basically, we grew up on what my parents prepared for us."

"Food practices are handed down from generation to generation. Once your body gets used to a particular type of food, it is not easy to switch to another type."

"Blacks eat spicer and fried food." (Airhihenbuwa et al. 1996: 251)

For theme no. 2 (context in which food is eaten), two primary domains probed in relation to the context of eating were preferences for eating in a restaurant versus at home and attitudes about with whom one eats or shares food. A majority felt more comfortable at home because there was more togetherness and less need to worry about table manners and about the cleanliness of the food prepared in the restaurant. Other reasons for preferring to eat at home involved not having to be watched by strangers when one eats and being able to relax better at home. The belief that there was a tendency to overeat in the restaurant and this could be harmful to persons on diets was also expressed (Airhihenbuwa et al. 1996: 252).

For theme no. 3 (healthfulness of soul food and other traditional food practices), probes related to traditional food practices included explicit questions about the definition, meaning, and health effects of soul food. Participants indicated that soul food consisted of using spices, cooking food thoroughly, and selecting fresh meat and vegetables and cooking them from scratch. The composition of soul food was thought to be influenced by slavery, economics, and discrimination. Participants made the following comments:

> *"Soul food consists of the way you cook it. You take like your green vegetables—we as blacks cook our green vegetables different than whites."*

> *"It's called soul food because it's associated with blacks; soul food is identified as those foods that are generally used by black folks and prepared in that fashion. I would identify soul food as home fries, compared to French fries, or deep fried chicken compared to baked chicken."*

> *"We ate basic things, chicken, fatback, beans, chitlins, a lot of poor homemade stuff like bread, ham, grits, fruit, vegetables and stuff like that."* (Airhihenbuwa et al. 1996: 253)

Airhihenbuwa et al. (1996) concluded that the food preferences and eating patterns commonly described for African Americans were easily elicited from these focus group participants as characteristic of soul food or the way African Americans eat. Many of these foods and food preparation practices have their roots in the history of the U.S. Southeast and are identical to those associated with the Southern dietary pattern (Airhihenbuwa et al. 1996: 256). The section that follows highlights the early beginnings of African American cuisine. In other words, *how soul food got its start!*

Cultural History of African American Cuisine

Before Emancipation (1600s–1864)

African Americans are primarily descendants of West African people who share a common history, place of origin, language, values, health beliefs, and food preferences that engender a sense of exclusiveness and self-awareness of being a member of this ethnic group (Staples 1971; Franklin and Moss 1988). As early as the 1500s, West Africans were forcibly transported to South America, the Caribbean, and North America. More than half of the West Africans came from the coastal areas of what are now Angola and Nigeria. Others came from the regions that are today Senegal, Gambia, Sierra Leone, Liberia, Togo, Ghana, Benin, Gabon, and Zaire. In addition, they belonged to different kinship groups—the Mandingo, Hausa, Efiks, Fanting, Ashanti, Bambara, Fulani, Ibo, Malinke, or Yoruba—and spoke different languages (Dixon and Wilson 1994: 17). In the process of adapting to the new settings, West Africans merged their African cultural traditions with European and Native American traditions.

Historically, even before West Africans were brought to the United States, their food habits had changed significantly due to the introduction of New World foods such as cassava (*Manihot esculenta,* a tuber that is also called *manioc*), corn, chiles, peanuts, pumpkins, and tomatoes during the fifteenth and sixteenth centuries (Kittler and Sucher 2000: 183). The slaves brought a cuisine based on these new foods and native West African foods, such as watermelon, black-eyed peas, okra, sesame, and taro. Adaptations and substitutions were made based on what foods were available. Black cooks added their West African preparation methods to British, French, Spanish, and Native American techniques to produce American Southern cuisine, emphasizing fried, boiled, and roasted dishes using pork, pork fat, corn, sweet potatoes, and green leafy vegetables (Kittler and Sucher 2000: 183).

Kittler and Sucher (2000) state that the diet of the African American slave field workers was largely dependent on whatever foods the slave owners provided. Salt pork and corn were the most common items. Sometimes rice (instead of corn), salted fish, and molasses were included. Greens, legumes, milk, and sweet potatoes were occasionally added. The foods provided, as well as their amount, were usually contingent on local availability and agricultural surplus (Kittler and Sucher 2000: 186). If slaves were allowed to maintain garden plots, okra and cow peas from Africa were favored, as well as American cabbage, collard and mustard greens, sweet potatoes, and turnips. Furthermore, during the hog-slaughtering season in the fall, a variety of pork cuts, such as chitterlings (intestines; pronounced *chitlins*), maw (stomach lining), tail, and hocks, would sometimes be given to slaves. Chicken, a prestigious food in West Africa, continued to be reserved for special occasions.

As the African slaves forcibly became more acclimated to their New World setting, the West African cooking methods were adapted to slave conditions. Boiling and frying remained the most popular ways to prepare not only meats but also vegetables and legumes. Bean stews maintained popularity as main dishes. Corn was substituted for most West African regional staple starches and was prepared in many forms, primarily as cornmeal pudding, cornmeal breads known as *pone* or *spoon bread*, grits (coarsely ground cornmeal), and *hominy* (hulled, dried corn kernels with the bran and germ removed). Pork fat (lard) replaced palm oil in cooking and was used to fry or flavor everything from breads to greens. Hot pepper sauces were used instead of fresh peppers for seasoning. No substitutions were available for many of the nuts and seeds used in West African recipes, although peanuts and sesame seeds remained popular (Kittler and Sucher 2000: 186).

Kittler and Sucher (2000) note that the diet for slave field workers was slightly different for the slaves who cooked in the homes of slave owners. For example, food for the slave field workers had to be portable. One-dish vegetable stews were common, as were fried cakes, such as *hushpuppies* (perhaps named because they were used to quiet whining dogs), and the cornmeal cakes baked in the fire on the back of a hoe, called *hoecakes.*

Slaves who cooked in the homes of slave owners, however, enjoyed a much more ample and varied diet. They popularized chicken and fried fish. They introduced "sticky" vegetable-based stews (thickened with okra or the herb sassafras, which when ground is called "file powder"), such as the Southern specialty *gumbo z'herbes.* Green leafy vegetables (called "greens") became a separate dish instead of being added to stews, but they were still cooked for hours and flavored with meat. Ingredients familiar to West Africans were used for pie fillings, such as nuts, beans, and squash (Kittler and Sucher 2000: 187).

After Emancipation (1865–1900)

One might think that finding out what African Americans consumed during this period of time would be more than impossible, yet quite interestingly there were major studies being conducted on food consumption in the United States. Systematically collected information began to appear in the 1880s when chemists became interested in nutritional requirements and how much food people consumed. W.O. Atwater, head of the USDA's Office of Experiment Stations (OES), took the lead in documenting American eating habits. He and his associates conducted field studies (Dirks and Duran 2001: 1881).

Atwater's colleagues selected family households, boarding houses, institutional dining halls, and other venues and groups regarded as typical of some region or segment of society. Atwater's method involved weighing all of the food on hand and everything entering the home for at least a week. Fieldworkers calculated the quantity consumed by deducting waste from the total weight. They also subtracted food remaining at the end of the study. Reports usually contained a brief description of household members and their activities. Authors provided a detailed list of the foods consumed and a nutritional analysis of each. Costs were recorded using prices at the nearest market for items home produced (Dirks and Duran 2001: 1881).

Atwater and his colleagues' fieldwork produced 49 studies involving African American households. Major projects conducted in Alabama and Virginia accounted for 5 of 39 of these. The rest were collected in the course of broader investigations in Philadelphia and Washington, D.C. There were also data from 60 students who boarded at the Institute for Colored Youth in Cheyney, Pennsylvania, and 20 individual African American women in New York City (Dirks and Duran 2001: 1881).

For example, Atwater's Tuskegee Alabama study that began in spring 1895 and completed in February 1896 included mostly tenant farmers and plantation workers with some villagers. Examination of their food consumption and pattern are as follows:

- Most popular form of pork was bacon.
- Eating fresh meat was rare.
- Families prepared simple meals.
- Bacon grease was mixed with molasses to make sap.

Atwater followed up his Tuskeege study with two projects in Eastern Virginia. In the first study, Atwater researched the eating habits of families living around the Great Dismal Swamp in Franklin County; and the second dealt with families in Elizabeth City County and the town of Hampton. Examination of their food consumption and pattern are as follows:

- Diets included considerable quantities of fish, but pork was eaten more.
- Fresh meat was seldom eaten.
- Fresh dairy foods were not eaten regularly.
- Children drank buttermilk.

Finally, researchers collected data from African American households in Philadelphia and Washington, D.C., as part of larger studies. The work in Philadelphia took place in 1892 and Washington, D.C., in summer 1905 and winter 1906. Examination of their food consumption and pattern are as follows:

- Beef, pork, and pork sausage were the most favored meats.
- Potatoes and sweet potatoes were consumed regularly.
- Cabbage was eaten often.

In general, from the three major studies along with the smaller sampled studies (60 students at the Institute of Colored Youth [now Cheyney University] and 20 African American women in New York City), Dirks and Duran (2001) state that these earliest systematic studies of eating habits represent a spectrum of typical African American diets at the beginning of the twentieth century. At one end, there are the "hog and hominy" traditions of the rural South and at the other end stands the respectable middle-class menu in which beef outranked pork and wheat was favored over corn. Interestingly, the sweet potato alone found a home everywhere. More than side meat and cornbread, it occupied an important place from the cotton lands of the Black Belt to the projects of Philadelphia (Dirks and Duran 2001: 1887).

Other Southern favorites appeared regularly on the tables of African Americans living in Philadelphia and Washington's projects. Pork sausage, rice, beans, and cabbage rated as core items. These same foods typically amounted to secondary or peripheral foods among poor urban whites. Bacon was part of the secondary core for blacks, but it was not a favorite of whites. Ham, chicken, cornmeal, hominy, and peanuts occupied the periphery of the urban diet of blacks (Dirks and Duran 2001: 1887).

Overall, we think of these foods as important components of the soul food tradition. As such, they represent Southern roots and African American ancestral experience. Interestingly, the African American cuisine that was developed and adapted before Emancipation and after Emancipation reflect the type of society that we had to live in; where we lived; under what circumstances; and it shows our tenacity in finding a way to survive in the most difficult situations. This is how "soul food" really got its start.

Contemporary Food Habits

Most researchers have noted that the food habits of African Americans today usually reflect their current socioeconomic status, geographic location, and work schedule more than their African or Southern heritage (Kittler and Sucher 2001: 192). African Americans throughout the country now eat lighter breakfasts and sandwiches at a noontime lunch. Dinner is served after work, and it has become the biggest meal of the day. Snacking throughout the day is still typical among most African Americans. In many households, meal schedules are irregular and family members eat when convenient. It is not unusual for snacks to replace a full meal.

Now that we have a better understanding of African American food habits, their beginnings, and the circumstances that influenced the type of foods being consumed and prepared a certain way, we also have a better understanding of what constitutes "soul food." So let's clearly define what soul food is and what type of foods are now considered soul food.

Soul Food Defined

As Tony Whitehead describes in his book chapter "In Search of Soul Food and Meaning: Culture, Food, and Health," historically, African American foodways are products of:

- African foods brought by the slave ships, and foods and other components of the African foodways created by the African servants

- Sociocultural processes that resulted in the integration of African, European, and Native American foodway systems

- A rural physical environment that has long supported traditional African and European foods that are now a part of the Southern food system

- Persistent economic and political marginality for African Americans

- The emergence of social, ideational, and organic (taste) preferences for patterns related to traditional Southern foodways

- The universal tendency for foodways to meet human needs other than mere nutrition. (Whitehead 1992: 101)

In otherwords, soul food is directly related to the food preferences and the types of foods available to the newly arrived enslaved Africans and later free African Americans of the past.

The soul food diet includes various uses of corn and sweet potatoes (including cornbread, grits, hominy, and sweet potato pudding and pie). Corn is frequently the base of numerous quick breads, hushpuppies (fried cornbread dough), johnnycake, dodgers, and hoecakes and is used in the frying of a traditional favorite: fish. Older African Americans of Southern roots would also include various wild game in the soul food menu, such as squirrel, rabbit, possum, and deer (Whitehead 1992: 98).

Whitehead (1992) also states that soul food is a reference not only to the content of the Southern African American diet but also to its *preparation styles*. Pork is a favorite soul food meat that must be fixed in a certain way. In addition, soul food requires the use of pork fat ("fatback," salt pork, streak-o-lean) as a seasoning in the cooking of vegetables in a slow, stewing manner (vegetables such as collard and turnip greens, black-eyed and field peas, green and lima beans), and in the frying of other favorite foods such as chicken, fish, and potatoes (Whitehead 1992: 98).

African Americans in the South have traditionally favored foods that were prepared with high contents of sugar or salt, as well as those that were "spiced up" with hot peppers, sauces such as Tabasco, and spices such as mace, allspice, sesame seed (called "beene"), and "file powder" (made from sassafras leaves). Northerners often remark that Southerners tend to prefer overly sweet desserts and summer drinks (lemonade, Quill-Acid, iced tea) (Whitehead 1992: 98).

Whitehead (1992) reminds us that soul food is more than just the type of specific foods associated with Africans and African Americans, it also involves the *preparation styles* of these foods. Whether it is cooking foods in a slow stewing manner, or frying, or even spicing up foods with sugar, salt, or peppers, soul food is a special taste and flavor with foods that have a lot of history.

The following is a list of traditional black core foods that are associated with soul food:

- Pig tails/ears/feet/heads/backs
- Head/backbones
- Kidney
- Chitterlings
- Fatback/salt pork/sidemeat
- Chicken wings/necks/backs/feet
- Collard/mustard/turnip greens
- Okra
- Sweet potatoes
- Corn
- Cornbread
- Pies/cakes/cookies
- Grits
- Buttermilk
- Tea
- Jelly/jams/preserves
- Neckbones
- Liver
- Brains
- Hamhocks
- Wild game
- Fish
- Cabbages
- Peas and beans
- White potatoes
- Poke salad
- Biscuits
- Rice
- Whole milk
- Coffee
- Onions
- Molasses

(Whitehead 1992: 102)

Now that we have defined soul food, highlighted its preparation, and listed some traditional black food types, it is time to review this African American cuisine in its broader context as it relates to the functions of food and food habits within African American culture.

Soul Food Cookbooks

One of the best ways to capture how black people feel about soul food is to do a survey of some of the popular soul food cookbooks of today and highlight some of their classic soul food cuisines. By doing this, you will begin to get a sense of how soul food has become a part of the African American experience and you will also begin to get a sense of why it may be very difficult for some to change their dietary eating pattern, particularly when soul food plays such an important part of our lives.

Soul Food Cookbook No. 1

For example, Joyce White's book *Soul Food: Recipes and Reflections from African American Churches* offers more than 150 recipes for the foods that worshippers look forward to after services, and she captured the spirit of these sociable meals with warm, conversational, and occasionally poignant reflections from African American churchgoers around the United States. White (1998) describes her book as follows:

> *"The recipes are varied and imaginative, and they reflect a much wider world than the one we lived in years ago. Today we add mushrooms to Grandma's smothered chicken and proclaim the dish fancy. One day we cook peas and rice or rice and beans and call it West Indian, and the next time we call it Hoppin' John, a dish that originated during slavery in the kitchens of the Carolinas and Georgia."*

> *"When company comes we fix gumbo or jambalaya or West African Jollof. Or we maybe stir up a pot of beans and rice and pork with chopped collard greens on the side, like our Brazilian soul sisters and brothers, and enjoy feijoada, their homeland's national dish. And when we cook at church we take all these inventive recipes with us, and they all reflect the culinary genius of the people of the African diaspora."* (White 1998: 4)

Soul Food Cookbook No. 2

Another soul food cookbook that captures the essence of how black people feel about food is by Sylvia Woods and Family, *Sylvia's Family Soul Food Cookbook: From Hemingway, South Carolina to Harlem*. Sylvia Woods, chef and owner of Sylvia's Restaurant on Lenox Avenue in Harlem, New York City, is celebrated around the world for her delicious, authentic, and satisfying soul food. In her cookbook, Sylvia has gathered more than 125 soul food classics, including recipes for okra, collard greens, Southern-style pound cakes, hearty meat and seafood stews and casseroles, salads, mashed potatoes, macaroni and cheese, and more. These recipes are straight from the heart of the Woods community of family and friends (Woods 1999).

For example, Sylvia Wood (1999) recalls that her mother made the best fried chicken in all of South Carolina and relates her mother's secrets to making it crunchy on the outside but keeping it tender on the inside. She would always shake the chicken in the coating, never dredge it. Then she cooked the chicken in a deep layer of oil in a black iron pan.

JOYCE WHITE'S OLD FASHIONED CORNBREAD

For centuries, one of the classic breads made among African Americans has been cornbread. Here is Joyce White's recipe for old fashioned cornbread:

2 cups yellow cornmeal	*1 tablespoon sugar*
½ cup all-purpose flour	*1 large egg*
¼ teaspoon salt	*1 to 1¼ cup milk*
¼ cup vegetable oil or shortening	*2½ teaspoons baking powder*

Preheat the oven to 425 degrees. Oil a 9-inch square or round pan; place to warm in the oven at least 5 minutes. In the meantime, sift into a medium bowl the cornmeal, flour, salt, baking powder, and sugar. Add the egg, vegetable oil or shortening, and milk and beat vigorously for 30 seconds. Carefully remove the hot pan from the oven. Pour in the cornmeal batter and shake the pan to level the batter. Set the pan in the oven on the lower shelf. Bake the bread about 25 minutes or until golden brown and puffy and a knife comes out clean when inserted into the center. Remove the pan from the oven and let the cornbread rest for a few minutes before cutting into wedges. Serve hot.

Joyce White describes her cornbread as "our staff of life" because it could be quickly made with little effort, it was a filling meal in itself when eaten with a baked sweet potato and a glass of cold buttermilk, and it could be eaten every day (White 1998: 8).

Sylvia elaborates further about the fried chicken her mother made:

"Fried chicken was a dish that she made for holidays and oftentimes for Sunday dinner. She also fried up a batch before sending the children anywhere by train, since fried chicken makes the most delicious sandwiches imaginable. She would put the chicken between two slices of white bread, which were covered with mayonnaise. The longer the chicken sandwiches

Sylvia Wood's Southern Fried Chicken

Here is Sylvia Wood's recipe for Southern fried chicken:

One 3½ pound chicken, cut into eighths

½ teaspoon garlic powder

1½ teaspoon salt

½ cup all-purpose flour

1¼ teaspoon freshly ground black pepper

¼ teaspoon paprika

1 cup vegetable oil

Rinse the chicken and pat dry. In a small bowl, combine the salt, 1 teaspoon of the black pepper, and the garlic powder. Sprinkle over the chicken. Let stand at least 20 minutes or, even better, overnight in the refrigerator. Place the flour, the remaining ¼ teaspoon black pepper, and paprika into a plastic bag. Add the seasoned chicken and shake until each piece is covered with the flour. In a large skillet, heat the oil over high heat until it bubbles when a little flour is sprinkled in. Add the chicken pieces and reduce the heat to medium. Cook for 7 to 10 minutes or until the chicken is nicely browned on the bottom. Turn and cook on the other side for 7 to 10 minutes or until cooked through. Remove from the skillet and drain on paper towels before serving.

sat, the better they tasted, since the crumblings from the chicken skin and the mayonnaise would soak into the soft white bread. My son, Kenneth, would sometimes just eat the bread by itself before eating the chicken, since it tasted so good. The sandwiches were packed into a shoebox with some fruit and maybe a piece of cake or pie. You were supposed to wait until lunchtime to eat the chick sandwiches, but none of the kids could ever wait that long." (Woods 1999: 82)

Soul Food Cookbook No. 3

The last soul food cookbook that I want to highlight here is Patti LaBelle's *LaBelle Cuisine: Recipes to Sing About. LaBelle Cuisine* is a book in which singer, diva Patti LaBelle invites you to her kitchen and serves up more than 100 of her favorite recipes, from treasured down-home favorites such as Say-My-Name Smothered Chicken and Gravy, Fierce Fried Corn, and

PATTI LABELLE'S BABYBACK RIBS

Here is Patti's recipe for babyback ribs. She calls them "Burnin' Babyback Ribs:"

4 pound babyback pork ribs	*1½ cups cider vinegar*
4 quarts water, approximately	*4 teaspoons salt*
2 cups Bodacious Barbecue Sauce	*Freshly ground black pepper*

Patti adds a tip to this babyback rib recipe:

"I always precook the ribs on the top of the stove to season and tenderize them before baking or grilling them with the sauce. Backyard cooks will love this method, as it cooks out most of the fat that usually drips down onto the fire and causes flare-up." (Labelle 1999: 44)

Aunt Hattie's Scrumptious Sweet Tater Bread to good-enough-for-dinner-parties dishes such as Shrimp Etouffee, Roast Leg of Lamb with Rosemary-Lemon Rub, and Aunt Mary's Philadelphia Buttercake (LaBelle 1999). Filled with the legendary diva's favorite dishes and step-by-step instructions on how to prepare them, *LaBelle Cuisine* makes you feel like Patti's in the kitchen with you, demonstrating the recipes and techniques that can turn anybody into a fabulous cook.

As Patti LaBelle (1999) states, her passion for food and cooking began when she was a little girl. In the very first paragraph of her book, she states,

> *"I knew there were two things in this world I was born to do: sing and cook. I've spent my life developing my voice and my recipes and, to tell you the truth, I'm hard pressed to say where I'm happiest— in concert or in the kitchen: making music and making meals. Whether cooking or singing, I feel at ease, at peace, at one with the world."* (Labelle 1999: xiii)

Interesting, if you notice in the examples of the aforementioned soul food cookbooks, each one of them showed a connection with their immediate family and their past family members when they expressed their joy and love for soul food. This past connection to their African American heritage and the manner in which soul food has remained a stable African American cuisine over the centuries is quite remarkable.

Conclusion

Research, cultural history and examples from the most recently published soul food cookbooks indicate that there is a pattern of similar food habits and eating patterns among African Americans. Earlier in this chapter, I highlighted several personal accounts of soul food and how it is expressed in the African American community. From Joyce White, to Sylvia Woods, and then to Patty LaBelle, you read their accounts on the importance of soul food to not only them but to their family and friends.

As Patty Labelle (1999) describes it:

> *"While reminiscing for this book, I realized why cooking has always been such a labor of love for me. Because it's as much about friendship and fellowship as it is about food. Because, behind the whole process – the shopping, the planning, the preparing, the serving – cooking is really about love. Cooking is a way to show it, share it, serve it. Cooking is as much about nourishment for the soul as it is the stomach."* (Labelle 1999: xiii)

Additionally, for Sylvia Woods (1999), soul food means "soul food and love are one and the same" (Woods 1999: 5); and finally, for Alexis Herman, soul food meant "homemade love" (National Council of Negro Women 1991: 39).

Postevaluation Questions

1. Should health professionals attempt to modify African Americans' food preferences?

    Health professionals should not initially modify African Americans' food preferences primarily because there is a wide array of cultural attachments to foods. However, once the opportunity presents itself and after the health professional has established a good rapport with the individual African American, then the health professional should definitely offer a wide variety of suggestions to modify food selection and food preparation among African Americans.

2. Are there strategies that health professionals can use to modify the dietary pattern of African Americans?

    Strategies that health professionals can use begin with spending quality time to listen and recognize the meaning and cultural connection that some African Americans have with their foods.

3. How can African Americans modify their traditional soul food dietary preferences in order to follow a healthier diet?

    African Americans can modify their traditional soul food dietary preferences to develop a healthier version by deciding to take small steps in selecting more health-conscious foods that are within their budgets, reducing the amounts of sodium and fat added to their meals, and asking a family member and/or friend to motivate them in modifying their dietary pattern.

References

Airhihenbuwa, C., Kumanyika, S., Agurs, T., Lowe, A., Saunders, D., and Morssink, C. 1996. Cultural aspects of African American eating patterns. *Ethnicity & Health* 1:245–260.

Dirks, R., and Duran, N. 2001. African American dietary patterns at the beginning of the 20th century. *Journal of Nutrition* 131:1881– 1889.

Dixon, B., and Wilson, J. 1994. *Good Health for African Americans*. New York: Crown Publishers.

Fieldhouse, P. 1992. *Food and nutrition: Customs and culture. Second Edition*. New York: Chapman & Hall.

Franklin, J., and Moss, A. 1988. *From Slavery to Freedom: A History of Negro Americans.* New York: Alfred A. Knopf.

Gary, T., Baptiste-Roberts, K., Gregg, E., Williams, D., Beckles, G., Miller, E., and Engelgau, M. 2004. Fruit, vegetable and fat intake in a population-based sample of African Americans. *Journal of the National Medical Association* 96(12):1599–1605.

Kittler, P., and Sucher, K. 2001. *Food and Culture.* Belmont, CA: Wadsworth Thomson Learning.

LaBelle, P. 1999. *LaBelle Cuisine: Recipes to Sing About.* New York: Broadway Books.

National Council of Negro Women. 1991. *The Black Family Reunion Cookbook.* New York: Fireside Book.

Neumark-Sztainer, D., Story, M., Hannan, P., and Croll, J. 2002. Overweight status and eating patterns among adolescents: Where do youths stand in comparison with the healthy people 2010 objectives. *American Journal of Public Health* 92:844–851.

Satia, J., Galanko, J., and Siega-Riz, A. 2004. Eating at fast-food restaurants is associated with dietary intake, demographic, psychosocial and behavioural factors among African Americans in North Carolina. *Public Health Nutrition* 7(8):1089–1096.

Schlundt, D., Hargreaves, M., and Buchowski, M. 2003. The eating behavior patterns questionnaire predicts dietary fat intake in African American women. *Journal of the American Dietetic Association* 103:338–345.

Staples, R. 1971. Towards a sociology of the black family: A theoretical and methodological assessment. *Journal of Marriage and Family* 33:19–138.

Whitehead, T. 1992. In search of soul food and meaning: Culture, food, and health. In H. Baer and Y. Jones (Eds.), *African Americans in the South: Issues of Race, Class and Gender.* Athens, GA: The University of Georgia Press, 94–110.

White, J. 1998. *Soul Food: Recipes and Reflections from African American Churches.* New York: Harper Collins.

Woods, S., and Family. 1999. *Sylvia's Family Soul Food Cookbook: From Hemingway, South Carolina, to Harlem.* New York: William Morrow and Company.

EXERCISE AND PHYSICAL FITNESS PERSPECTIVES AMONG AFRICAN AMERICANS

Critical Thinking Questions

1. Do African Americans have a different view of exercise and physical fitness than other Americans?
2. Why are there so few books targeted for African Americans in the area of exercise and physical fitness?
3. Do African Americans consider exercise and physical fitness important factors in losing weight?
4. Why is it difficult to get African Americans to adhere to an exercise and physical fitness regimen?

Introduction

There is no doubt that Americans are not physically active enough. Only 45 percent of adults get the recommended 30 minutes of physical activity on five or more days per week, and adolescents are similarly inactive (U.S. Department of Health and Human Services 2000; Centers for Disease Control and Prevention 2004). Regular physical activity improves aerobic capacity, muscular strength, body agility, and coordination (U.S. Department of Health and Human Services 1996). Those who are physically active have a reduced risk of cardiovascular disease, stroke, type 2 diabetes, colon cancers, osteoporosis, depression, and fall-related injuries (Paffenbarger, Hyde, and Wing 1984; Farmer et al. 1989; Nichols et al.

1994; Giovannucci et al. 1995; Fox 1999; Hu, Stampfer, and Colditz 2000; Hu et al. 2001).

Although it is almost common knowledge that physical activity and exercise are beneficial to one's health, there is a misunderstanding as to what constitutes physical activity, leisure-time physical activity, physical fitness, and exercise. According to the Centers for Disease Control and Prevention (2005), the public needs to be aware of these distinctions. Below are the definitions:

- **Physical activity** is defined as any bodily movement produced by skeletal muscles resulting in energy expenditure.

- **Leisure-time physical activity** is exercise, sports, recreation, or hobbies that are not associated with activities as part of one's regular job duties, household, or transportation.

- **Physical fitness** is a set of attributes a person has in regard to ability to perform physical activities that require aerobic fitness, endurance, strength, or flexibility and is determined by a combination of regular activity and genetically inherited ability.

- **Exercise** is a physical activity that is planned or structured. It involves repetitive bodily movement done to improve or maintain one or more of the components of physical fitness—cardiorespiratory endurance (aerobic fitness), muscular strength, muscular endurance, flexibility, and body composition. (Centers for Disease Control and Prevention 2005)

Overall, it is important to get a basic understanding of an individual's or a group's perspective of these concepts in order to find out how to begin a successful health-and-fitness program.

It is also important to be aware of some of the general U.S. patterns associated with physical activity. According to the Centers for Disease Control and Prevention (1996) and several research studies, patterns of physical activity vary with demographic characteristics:

- Men are more likely than women to engage in regular activity, in vigorous exercise, and in sports.

- The total amount of time spent engaging in physical activity declines with age.

- Adults at retirement age (65 years) show some increased participation in activities of light to moderate intensity, but, overall, physical activity declines continuously as age increases.

- People with higher levels of education participate in more leisure-time physical activity than do people with less education.

- Differences in education and socioeconomic status account for most, if not all, of the differences in leisure-time physical activity associated with race/ethnicity.

- African Americans and other ethnic minority populations are less active than white Americans. (Stephens, Jacobs, and White 1985; Schoenborn 1986; Stephens 1987; White et al. 1987; DiPietro and Caspersen 1991; Caspersen and Merritt 1992; Centers for Disease Control and Prevention 1996; Pate et al. 1995)

How Blacks Feel About Exercise

As described in the previous chapter on soul food and African Americans' food preferences, one of the best ways to gauge how blacks feel about workin' out and exercising is to review a few of the most popular nonfiction books targeted to the African American community with regard to exercise and fitness. Unfortunately, the list on exercise and fitness books targeted to the African American community is small. In fact, there are really only three to acknowledge.

First, I am going to highlight a book that is not directly related to exercise and fitness yet offers advice to others, particularly older African Americans, on the need for individuals to follow an exercise routine. The book is entitled *The Delany Sisters' Book of Everyday Wisdom*. Sarah and A. Elizabeth Delany took the reading public by storm in 1993 with their surprise bestseller *Having Our Say: The Delany Sisters' First 100 Years*. In a memoir that's as much a historical record as a testimony to two extraordinary women and sisters, they recall their remarkable lives, spanning more than a century of the African American experience. Since then, they decided to address all the questions about their lives in the book *The Delany Sisters' Book of Everyday Wisdom* (1994).

One major question that the Delany sisters were often asked: "What is your secret for living past 100 years?" They responded as follows:

> *"There's another thing I make Bessie do that she doesn't like too much, and that's exercise. You've got to exercise, not just*

for your heart and lungs, but to keep from stiffening up. It keeps you limber, and that's important when you get older."

"We started doing yoga about forty years ago, but don't think we didn't get exercise before that! When we were younger and lived in New York City, we'd walk for miles because we couldn't afford to take the trolley. That was mighty good exercise!

"You don't have to get down on the floor and do yoga. You can get exercise from doing housework, gardening, all kinds of things—anything's better than sitting on your behind all day long." (Delany, Delany, and Hearth 1994: 111)

The Delany sisters' comments show that even though they walked more when they were younger, they still followed an exercise routine in their later years.

Another book that is specifically targeted to African American women with a thorough exercise and fitness plan is *Slim Down Sister* (2000). *Slim Down Sister*, the first weight-loss book written especially for African American women, addresses the serious health concerns facing African American women today and offers a comprehensive, get-down-to-it program of diet and exercise that empowers sisters to take control of their weight and health. One topic that this book highlights is exercise. Specifically, exercises designed for African American women and their particular body type. Here are a few comments as to how they feel about workin' out:

"The bottom line is that you need to move your body if you want to lose weight—period. There's no two ways about it. Sure, you can probably drop a few pounds by drastically cutting your caloric intake. But sooner or later your body's going to rebel. And you know what that means. Those pounds are going to come back with a vengeance. Chances are, you'll end up weighing more than you did when you started out." (Weaver, Gains, and Ebron 2000: 45)

"So what's the key to revving up your engine, that is, your metabolism? You guessed it—exercise. Break a good sweat and your body won't be inclined to hang onto those calories at all costs. You'll burn them up, and not just during your workout. Research proves that vigorous exercise has an added bonus: afterburn. Your metabolism keeps running strong even after your workout is done, so you'll still be burning calories hours later. And that's good news for sisters like you who are ready to take charge of their health. (Weaver, Gains, and Ebron 2000: 46)

Slim Down Sister is one of those books that truly engages the African American woman in a style, dialogue, and approach that makes it so much easier for any African American woman regardless of background to take action about her weight, fitness, and exercise situation. We need more books like this one.

The third and final book that I would like to highlight is Madonna Grimes' *Work It Out: The Black Women's Guide to Getting the Body You Always Wanted* (2003). Fitness expert MaDonna Grimes offers black women a different ideal to work toward—one suited to their unique physiques. Drawing from her experience as a professional dancer, choreographer, fitness competitor, and winner of Miss Fitness America and Miss Fitness International competitions, Grimes (2003) has fashioned a fitness program specifically for black women, to help them attain their fitness goals and build self-esteem.

The major reason why Grimes (2003) wrote her book:

"I just got tired of watching women with beautiful shapely curves hold themselves up to impossible ideals and try to redesign their bodies into shapes that they were just never meant to be, leaving them like failures in the end. You know how good you can look. Enhance your curves; don't lose them." (Grimes 2003: 1)

In her book, *Work It Out,* Grimes offers a simple plan to allow the individual to be consistent when it comes to building and maintaining his or her body. Her integration of dance and weight training along with dieting is designed to transform your body and also to provide permanent weight loss (Grimes 2003: 3). She states:

"The first step of your weight training is, believe it or not, cardio. You've got to engage in twenty to thirty minutes of some kind of cardio exercise to warm up your muscles. You can go with either the treadmill or the stationary bike; both will burn calories while elevating your heart rate to its target range."

"Personally, I love doing my cardio on a treadmill. It works you harder than the bike. You can incline the treadmill to make it even more challenging. And, of course, you get all the same electronic programs for motivation that go with the stationary bike." (Grimes 2003: 63)

Grimes further states that step two of the weight-training program is the actual weight training.

"I'm telling you that this workout should not last more than thirty minutes. What's the point of wasting precious time? I want you in and out of the gym with the best possible outcome for your time invested. Unless I say otherwise for a specific exercise, start with the minimum comfortable weight, and over time as it gets easier to lift that weight, work your way up in 10-pound increments." (Grimes 2003: 63–64)

Surprisingly, *Work It Out* is one of the first health and fitness books designed specifically for African American women by an African American woman fitness expert. Grimes completes this groundbreaking book with the following parting message:

"Sister are doing it themselves. But we still have to keep the faith and live the life that brings emotional well-being, spiritual fulfillment, and a healthy, sexy body to be proud of." (Grimes 2003: 126)

Research Studies on Physical Fitness and African Americans

There is little doubt that the U.S. public health system and U.S. public health officials are quite well aware of Americans' lack of physical fitness and regular exercise. In fact, former U.S. Surgeon General Dr. David Satcher organized a national summit of health and education experts to discuss ways to trim the fat from young people (*USA Today* 2002). Additionally, Dr. Julie Gerberding, the director of the Centers for Disease Control and Prevention (CDC), and the scientists at CDC are trying different experiments to build fitness back into society—playing music to entice elevator users onto the stairs, starting walk-to-school programs, constructing sidewalks, and handing out pedometers.

As Dr. Benjamin Caballero of Johns Hopkins University in Baltimore stated:

"To reduce some of the main killers of America, we will have to increase the level of physical activity." (*USA Today* 2003)

Because physical activity, fitness, and exercise play a vital role not only in losing weight but also in reducing your chances of developing chronic diseases such as hypertension, cancer, stroke, and diabetes, we must examine the physical activity patterns among African Americans and find out which fitness and exercise regimen truly works in all types of African American communities.

African American Adolescent Studies

Perhaps one of the states that is an indicator for a number of social, cultural, and health trends in the United States is the state of California. Recently, a report from the UCLA Center for Health Policy Research stated that many California teens do not get regular physical activity or get no activity at all. Teenage girls, teens from low-income families, teens with no access to safe parks or open spaces, teens whose schools do not require physical education, and Latino, Asian, and African American teens are particularly at risk (Babey et al. 2005).

According to the data from the 2003 California Health Interview Survey, the researchers found the following major results:

- Teenage girls are less active than boys.

- Nearly three-quarters of boys (74.6%) participate in regular physical activity compared with only two-thirds of girls (66.5%).

- Girls have a higher prevalence of inactivity than boys (9.2% vs. 5.5%).

- Inactivity among teenage girls has nearly doubled to 9.2 percent in 2003 from 2001 when 5 percent of girls got no physical activity.

- Teens from low-income families are less active than more affluent teens.

- Latino (68.1%), Asian (62.3%), and African American teens (62.7%) report lower rates of regular physical activity than white teens (76.4%).

- The proportion of Latino (9.5%) and African American teens (12.3%) getting no physical activity is two to three times higher than white teens. (Babey et al. 2005: 2–3)

Although there are a variety of factors that contribute to the disparity in physical activity between the various groups, the researchers highlighted two major factors: (1) lack of safe parks and open spaces, and (2) lack of physical education in schools (Babey et al. 2005: 3). In order to reduce this disparity and increase physical activity among adolescents, particularly among African American, Latinos, and Asians, the researchers suggest that the state of California should focus on assuring increased opportunities at school and more safe opportunities out of school. Investing state and community resources in creating safe and accessible environments is important to making regular physical activity a lifelong pattern for all Californians (Babey et al. 2005).

Another study that I want to highlight among African American adolescents is a qualitative study entitled "Influences on Diet and Physical Activity among Middle-Class African American 8- to 10-Year-Old Girls at Risk of Becoming Obese." Researchers conducted interviews and group qualitative discussions among 8- to 10-year-old African American girls and their parents in the greater Houston metropolitan area to understand diet, physical activity, and inactivity influences among preadolescent African American girls at risk of becoming obese (Thompson et al. 2003).

Qualitative research methods were employed to facilitate in-depth exploration of influences on children's diet and physical activity practices. Most sessions were held Saturday mornings at the Children's Nutrition Research Center because this was the time and location that families reported most convenient for them. Staff who conducted the focus groups had conducted previous focus group discussions, read through the questionnaires in role-playing sessions, and thoroughly discussed issues that arose in this role-playing. Transcribed notes were used for analysis (Thompson et al. 2003: 116–117).

Qualitative analysis of the in-depth interviews and focus groups centered upon (1) influences on diet and (2) influences on physical activity and inactivity. In particular, with regard to influences on physical activity and inactivity, for 8- to 10-year-old African American girls to be more physically active, daughters and their parents suggested a broad variety of "fun activities," for example, "swimming," "play sports like soccer, basketball," "bike riding," "skating," and "jumping rope" (Thompson et al. 2003: 119).

Most girls reported that they were worried that they were not physically active enough. Busy schedules, homework, "smelling like a boy," and television prevented them from becoming more physically active. In addition, girls mentioned preference for indoor activities and not wanting to feel tired as reasons that they would not want to be physically active. According to girls, getting hurt was the most often mentioned "bad thing" that could happen because of exercise (Thompson et al. 2003: 119).

Parents, however, believed that their daughters did not think much about being physically active, even those who reported having highly active daughters. Many parents with concerns for their daughters' weights reported that they often encouraged physical activity and expressed those concerns to their daughters. Nevertheless, most parents felt that their daughters had high self-esteem:

> *"She says that she knows that she is a little thick around the waist but she likes herself. But she wishes she wasn't so thick."* (Thompson et al. 2003: 120)

When asked about parental/child exercise, most daughters reported that they were active with their siblings and/or father. Although one daughter reported that her mother was her basketball team's coach, mothers' participation in their daughters' physical activity tended to be on weekends as a spectator of their daughters' team sports. Some parents were involved with daughters in walking and low-impact fitness videotapes. One daughter said of the overall tone of parental physical activity participation:

"My mom is classical kind of. She's an indoor person. My dad is an outdoor person. He takes me camping ... fishing ... to tennis ... swimming." (Thompson et al. 2003: 120)

Moreover, most parents reported that their daughters like physical education. Although some daughters liked physical education, they disliked the running, individual or isolated activities such as jumping rope alone, or sitting out.

"I hate running laps in front of the hot sun. Some of my friends are ... always ahead of us. The rest of us feel tired and exhausted." (Thompson et al. 2003: 120)

Overall, this is the first research to have examined the influences on dietary intake and physical activity among 8- to 10-year-old middle-class African American girls. The researchers contend that contrary to earlier reports, there is substantial concern for overweight at least among some middle-class African American families. A study by Gordon-Larsen et al. (2004) found similar concerns among African American families. This concern could provide a motivational substrate for intervention but will need to be approached cautiously given the known sensitivities to the label "obese" and "overweight." To avoid offensively targeting the "overweight" or "obese" population, programs could be offered to volunteer responders to advertisements (Thompson et al. 2003:120; Ward, D., Trost, S., Felton, G., Saunders, R., Parsons, M., Dowda, M., and R. Pate. 1997).

African American Women Studies

In a study entitled "Physical Activity in Urban White, African American, and Mexican American Women," researchers analyzed physical activity in a diverse sample of urban women relative to race/ethnicity, income, age, and education, using a sex-specific questionnaire (Ransdell and Wells 1998). They also wanted to determine: (1) which demographic and anthropometric factors were predictive of high or low leisure-time physical activity (LTPA), energy expenditure (EE), and (2) how many of the women met the minimum requirements for physical activity as suggested by the

Surgeon General (i.e., moderate to vigorous physical activity most days of the week for a minimum of 30 minutes).

Subjects were drawn from a convenience sample of urban Phoenix women (n = 521) between the ages of 16 and 85 (mean 42.3 years). Most of the white women were recruited from professional women's organizations, businesses, Arizona State University, and a city government office. African American and Mexican American women were recruited primarily from local health fairs and churches. Before participating in the study, subjects completed an informed consent form according to procedures by Arizona State University (Randsell and Wells 1998: 1609).

The major results of the study indicated that the majority of the urban Phoenix women in this study were physically inactive and expended most of their kilocalories in light activity. Specifically, 62 percent of the minority women and 54 percent of the white women had no leisure-time physical activity. Additionally, women of color, women over 40, and those without a college degree were least likely to be highly active in leisure-time physical activity and most likely to be sedentary. Therefore, these results indicate that public health efforts to increase physical activity in women should be focused on women of color, women over 40, and women without a college degree (Ransdell and Wells 1998: 1614).

In another study that investigated African American women, researchers explored African American women's experiences with physical activity in their daily lives. The study, entitled "African American Women's Experiences with Physical Activity in their Daily Lives," involved women aged 35–50 years, healthy, employed and unemployed, at self-reported middle- to low-income level and living in an urban area (Nies, Vollman, and Cook 1999). Two focus groups with a total of sixteen women were conducted to obtain information from African American women about their experiences with facilitators and barriers to exercise in their daily lives.

The focus groups were held at a community clinic convenient for the women. Permission to tape-record the session and informed consent were obtained before beginning the session. The focus groups were led by an African American nurse who held a master's degree and who had been trained by the principal investigator as the group facilitator. The women were encouraged to ask questions during the sessions. Discussions were audio-recorded and transcribed verbatim for analysis (Nies, Vollman and Cook 1999: 25).

The major facilitator themes that emerged during analysis for African American women included: (a) daily routine, (b) practical and convenient activities, (c) personal safety, (d) child care, (e) weight loss, (f) stress reduction, (g) knowledge and commitment, (h) enjoyment, (i) pets, (j) family and peer support, (k) home and work facilities, and (l) daylight and climate conditions. Comments from the African American women on each of the major facilitator themes are as follows:

Daily Routine: *"The only exercise I really get is first thing in the morning ... I walk from home to the bus stop."*

Practical and Convenient Activities: *"I don't exercise that often, but when I do have time I walk around the building with my children and go to the park and play with them. I want something that I can do every day, but not too long."*

Personal Safety: *"I just need somebody to go with me (to exercise), because it is so dangerous at night."*

Child Care: *"My biggest hassle is child care while I'm working out. A free babysitter is at the top of my list. As long as I had a babysitter, it wouldn't matter what time I exercised. If I had to take my kids to exercise, I would need a place there that I could keep them."*

Weight Loss: *"I want to do the type of exercise that helps me get toned and make me lose some inches."*

Stress Reduction: *"I think talking with somebody (during exercise) about what actually happened during the day takes a lot of the stress off."*

Knowledge and Commitment: *"I think that would help a lot of women if they knew the importance of exercise. Some people know and still have a problem, but maybe if someone told them how important exercise was to them (they would take it more seriously)."*

Enjoyment: *"I like exercising. After the kids leave, I do it (exercise) because I enjoy that music and because I like dancing. I think I found my niche."*

Pets: *"Running after the dog ... you get your exercise."*

Family and Peer Support: *"We like the idea of exercising (together) and we knew that there was going to be more than one person there so that's a group environment. I went (to exercise class) religiously because there were people there."*

Home and Work Facilities: *"All I have is the floor, the rug, and the TV. You can exercise all day long. You have the upstairs, so you can go up and down. You know, having an 8- and 10-year-old helps ... running after them."*

Daylight and Climate Conditions: *"When the weather is nice, I can leave my house and go to the fairgrounds and I walk about two miles ... and we do that about every day we have enough daylight. You can walk three miles before you know it, and you really feel good ... you feel like you can do anything."* (Nies, Vollman, and Cook 1999: 25–28)

On the opposite end, the major barriers that emerged during analysis for African American women included: (a) lack of child care, (b) no person to exercise with, (c) competing responsibilities, (d) lack of space in the home, (e) inability to use exercise facilities at work, (f) lack of understanding and motivation, (g) fatigue, and (h) unsafe neighborhood. The one comment that reflects African American womens' barrier to exercising is as follows:

> *"But if exercise is by yourself, I'm not motivated. Without the structure I won't do it. Exercise is like way down on the bottom of my list; oh, I'll do it tomorrow. I'm a procastinator; I had my first heart attack and I'm supposed to ride a bike, but to be truthful I do it very seldom."* (Nies, Vollman, and Cook 1999: 29)

In conclusion, Nies, Vollman, and Cook's study (1999) found that the dominant factor that influenced the role of physical activity in the lives of African American women was the identification of practical, convenient, and enjoyable forms of exercise that can be performed routinely. As a result, these African American women reported identifying creative ways to incorporate physical activity into their routine activities such as work and household obligations.

The role of social support for physical activity also was identified by African American woman as an important facilitator of physical activity in their daily lives. Moreover, findings suggest that African American women understand the value of exercise in their daily lives.

These findings suggest that health promotion efforts should include the following components: develop approaches that use a family context including: family pets; personal and neighborhood safety; support mechanisms at home and work; and child care. Approaches that increase knowledge levels, offer appropriate support models, and provide positive experiences will be essential for improving the exercise behavior of African American women (Nies, Vollman, and Cook 1999: 30).

Finally, in the study entitled "Motivations for Exercise and Weight Loss Among African American Women: Focus Group Results and Their Contribution Towards Program Development," Young et al. (2001) explored the major factors that motivate African American women to engage in regular physical activity and maintain weight loss. The predominant themes that provided the motivation for the current exercisers to maintain their exercise program was feeling good and having energy as a result of regular exercise. Here are some comments from the women:

> *"I'm motivated by the fact that I like to look good and feel good, I feel good, and I feel good when I exercise, I feel energized… I can constantly go, the motivating factor is that I feel good."*

> *"I feel a lot better and people do notice. Guys are looking, and I'm not going to rule that out, that helps, too."*

> *"I can see that it contributes in a lot of different ways. Managing stress, so it helps me physically, it helps me mentally, it helps me emotionally, it gives me the opportunity to take some time out for myself, which I don't do any other time, and maintaining the weight, staying healthier."* (Young et al. 2001: 234)

Older African Americans

Another study of physical activity among African Americans involved a study investigating attitudes and beliefs toward exercise among older African Americans. According to Lavizzo-Mourey et al. (2001), their findings may be important in designing effective exercise programs for older African Americans in urban settings.

The study, entitled "Attitudes and Beliefs about Exercise among Elderly African Americans in an Urban Community," was a qualitative study using focus group methodology to identify culturally determined attitudes that could be useful in designing effective exercise programs. Specifically, the study involved five focus groups that were convened during the months of July and August 1999. Focus group discussions included open-ended questions about daily activities, physical difficulties and challenges, exercise, and fear of falling, as well as views on enjoyable and feasible exercises (Lavizzo-Mourey et al. 2001: 475–476).

The four major focus group questions were as follows:

- What do you consider as exercise?
- What makes exercise difficult for you?
- How can exercise be helpful to you?
- What kinds of exercise would you like to do?

Analysis of findings from the focus groups revealed that the preferences for exercise by older African Americans differed from the preconceived notions of the investigative team. They had originally planned to limit the number of group-exercise sessions to minimize inconvenience, reduce costs of transportation, and ensure a private setting conducive to long-term adherence. They learned, however, that almost everyone in the focus groups preferred group exercise and, contrary to their expectations, embarrassment about sweating and exercising in co-ed groups were not perceived as significant (Lavizzo-Mourey et al. 2001: 479).

Another important finding was the level of concern about safety when walking in urban neighborhoods. As a result of this concern, the research team was forced to rethink the original plan for a walking program and substitute a home-based dancing activity. Because participants were not familiar with Eastern exercises, the research team elected to incorporate a few Tai Chi–like controlled movements into the exercise routine rather than focus on an intensive and comprehensive Tai Chi approach. Finally, Lazizzo-Mourey et al. (2001) suggested that preferences for group sessions, dancing, and minimal interest in using weights and Tai Chi may have reflected cultural differences that could be important in the future design of effective programs of exercise for older African Americans in urban communities.

Another study on older African Americans that I want to highlight is entitled "A Synthesis of Perceptions About Physical Activity Among Older African American and American Indian Women." Because of the lack of information about women of color and their health needs, the Centers for Disease Control and Prevention funded several projects in the 1990s to examine minority racial groups and their physical activity involvement. One project was initiated through the Prevention Research Center of the University of South Carolina School of Public Health. The Cross-Cultural Activity Participation Study (CAPS) was designed to measure the physical activity habits in a sample of African American and American Indian women to develop and validate a set of surveys to measure moderate physical activity. Part of the study was focused on measuring physical activity patterns through surveys, daily physical activity records, and mechanical devices (e.g., Caltrac energy expenditure measurement equipment, pedometers). In addition, 56 women (30 African American and 26 American Indian) participated in in-depth qualitative interviews. This qualitative component was included as part of the larger study to obtain additional information about the psychosocial context and sociocultural meanings of physical activity and leisure (Henderson and Ainsworth 2003: 313).

The major results from their qualitative analysis highlighted six themes: physical activity values, constraints, social support, sedentary but busy, sociocultural concerns, and enjoyment as reflected in walking. With regard to physical activity values, for example, most of the women interviewed believed that physical activity was important for physical and mental health reasons. Despite this attitude, many of the women indicated that they were not physically active on a regular basis. Both the African American and American Indian women associated being physically active with feeling good, being with others, being and feeling healthy, and experiencing spiritual and psychological benefits. One African American woman stated:

> *"I think that for me to be truly happy or satisfied, I'm going to have to be physically active."* (Henderson and Ainsworth 2003: 314)

The researchers also found out as they listened to the African American and American Indian women talk about their lives that they were involved with a vast number of activities. These women may be defined as "sedentary" by physical activity standards, but they were certainly busy. Most of the women in this study noted a clear differentiation between weekend and the weekday as evidenced by the different activities mostly pertaining to paid work in their lives. Although the time seemed to be more flexible on the weekend than during the week, physical activity for the most part was not a planned aspect of the weekend (Henderson and Ainsworth 2003: 315).

Finally, the researchers found that walking was an important activity in the lives of many of the African American and American Indian women because of the available contexts, the conditions that enabled it to happen, and the negotiability of many of the constraints. As many of these women stated, walking had value because it was "not really exercise" and that this activity involved choices (Henderson and Ainsworth 2003: 316).

In general, this study's findings provide some descriptive information about the lives of African American and American Indian women and their physical activity. In some cases, the experiences of African American and American Indian women were similar; in other situations, ethnic as well as individual differences were evident. The researchers emphasize that other researchers must continue to try to ascertain the perceptions that people hold about their lives and discover the most valid ways to examine the meanings that individuals and groups attach to their lives and the role physical activity plays in them (Henderson and Ainsworth 2003: 317).

Another similar study that I want to highlight is entitled "Older Adult Perspectives on Physical Activity and Exercise: Voices from Multiple Cultures." To better understand the needs and desires for physical activity programs among older, ethnic minority adults, the researchers conducted focus groups with older adults from seven cultural groups, including five groups of older immigrants. The purposes of the study were to: (1) identify barriers and facilitators to engaging in physical activity and (2) broaden their understanding of culturally appropriate physical activity and exercise programs (Belza et al. 2004).

Focus groups were conducted with older adults to explore the motivations and barriers to physical activity within each of seven cultural/linguistic groups: American Indian and Native Alaskan, African American, Vietnamese, Cantonese-speaking Chinese immigrants from Vietnam, Korean, Tagalog-speaking immigrants from the Philippines, and Spanish-speaking immigrants primarily from Mexico and also from El Salvador, Columbia, Nicaragua, Peru, and Equador. The focus groups were conducted in the primary languages of participants. Participants were recruited from local community agencies and represented large minority communities in the Seattle area, as well as groups that have been typically underserved by existing programs promoting physical activity. Four community agencies partnered with the university-based research team. These four community partners were social and health service providers that met the needs of the specific ethnic groups (Belza et al. 2004: 2).

Professional translators transcribed the audiotapes into the language of the group and then translated the transcript into English. QSR NVivo qualitative analysis software was used to organize the data. Members of the research team representing several disciplines, including cultural anthropology, nursing, social work, and public administration, systematically reviewed the translated transcripts, coding them for emerging themes. The team members had expertise in aging, exercise, and community-based participatory research (Belza et al. 2004: 3).

Major themes emerged after reading and discussing the transcripts, coding reports, and summaries. A draft report of the results was sent to facilitators, note takers, and other representatives from the partner agencies. The research team convened a meeting of community partners to elicit feedback on the draft results and to enrich the interpretation of findings, including ideas for potential programming (Belza et al. 2004: 3).

The research team found four common themes among the 7 groups and 71 older adults who participated in the study. The major themes were: (1) physical activity as health promotion, (2) complex role of chronic conditions, (3) family as encouragement, and (4) environmental barriers (Belza et al. 2004: 4).

As for the African Americans (6) who participated in the focus groups, the strongest theme from them was that of friends encouraging each other to be regularly active.

"It's nice to have a friend, because if you don't feel like going, she might say something to encourage you. Or she might be after you so much that you say, 'Oh, yeah, I'll go.' And you feel so much better afterwards. Believe me."

Participants also understood the current recommendation of exercising a total of 30 minutes a day in shorter cumulative intervals.

"You can walk for 30 minutes a day or go about five to 10 minutes, and then go back home, and later on do the same thing. I read this in a book."

Additionally, several participants spoke enthusiastically about determination:

"Main thing, you don't get lazy and you don't give up. You gotta have determination." (Belza et al. 2004: 4)

Overall, the results of this study revealed that although there are ethnic-specific variations in factors influencing physical activity, there are more common themes than variations. The researchers noted that although lack of health contributes to sedentary lifestyles, lack of health also serves as a motivator to become more physically active. Changes in health status, therefore, may serve as cues to adopt a healthier lifestyle. In contrast with other studies that explore barriers and enhancers to physical activity, this study found that certain factors, such as one's physical health, could serve as both barriers to and enhancers of physical activity (Belza et al. 2004: 6).

Urban African Americans

In a similar study, researchers assessed physical activity patterns in a large sample of urban African Americans. The study of Young et al. (1998) was part of a community-based nutrition and physical activity intervention conducted in East Baltimore, a community in which more than 85 percent of the residents are African American. Surveys were conducted during the health fairs arranged at the area churches. Twenty-eight churches were randomly selected from 250 predominately African American churches in the community. The majority (68%) of residents in East Baltimore attend a church, and churches access approximately 85 percent of the adult population in this community through religious services, soup kitchens, and social programs (Young et al. 1998: 100).

There were 743 individuals who participated in the health fairs; 251 women and 114 men were interviewed about their physical activity pattern. Questions regarding physical activity participation were added after the health fairs had commenced; hence, physical activity participation was assessed at only 19 of the 26 churches. The sample was primarily middle-aged, employed, and had at least a high school diploma (Young et al. 1998: 103).

The major results of the study were as follows:

- The majority of men (54%) and women (69%) reported participating in at least one leisure-time exercise or sport activity during the prior month.

- Brisk walking (26%) was the most commonly-reported activity.

- For men, 74 percent walked at a brisk pace for at least 30 minutes and 78 percent walked at least three times per week.

- For women, 66 percent walked at a brisk pace for at least 30 minutes and 87 percent walked at least three times per week.

- Men were more likely not to engage in any leisure-time physical activity.

- More than one-third of men and women who were employed reported that they spent more than half of their work day walking. (Young et al. 1998: 103–104)

In conclusion, this study suggests that, among African Americans attending church-based health fairs, participation in regular leisure-time activity was low. The majority, however, engaged in at least some physical activity in the prior month, and based on the study's composite definition (i.e., walking at least ten blocks to and from work, walking more than half the time on the job, or regular leisure-time activity), approximately 40 percent of the sample was active.

This study also found that walking is a well-accepted physical activity among African Americans in this age group (Young et al. 1998: 109). This cultural preference for walking becomes a place to start when clinicians and public health officials begin designing health intervention programs for local African American communities.

Three additional studies that used similar qualitative measures to collect data on the attitudes and beliefs about physical activity among African Americans and found similar results are "Motivations for Exercise and Weight Loss Among African American Women: Focus Group Results and Their Contribution towards Program Development" (Young et al. 2001); "Perceptions and Beliefs About Exercise, Rest, and Health among African Americans" (Airhihenbuwa et al. 1995); and "An Ecological Approach to Physical Activity in African American Women" (Walcott-McQuigg et al. 2001). These particular studies offer additional in-depth reasons on the major factors that contribute to African Americans' participation and lack of participation in physical fitness activity.

Similarly, the study entitled "Perceptions and Beliefs About Exercise, Rest, and Health Among African Americans" found that among its male and female African American sample, exercise was generally believed to contribute to a sense of well-being. Health problems that were thought to be potentially alleviated by exercise included tension, heart disease, hypertension, "fluid buildup," strokes, knee and ankle problems, arthritis, stiffness, fatigue, lung problems, diabetes, back strain, and pulled muscles (Airhihenbuwa et al. 1995: 428). Here are some comments from the men and women:

"I think exercise will help fatigue, because if you just sit on your butt all day, not doing nothing, you'll be easily more tired than if you actually do something."

"First you have to develop a mental exercise, because if your mind ain't set on exercising, then you won't push yourself to exercise physically."

"Culturally, the reason why blacks don't exercise as much as they do is because we haven't been exercising, we have other things to be concerned about." (Airhihenbuwa et al. 1995: 428)

Interestingly, each of these studies mentioned in this section and others that are yet to be published recognize that it is extremely important to find out:

- How do African Americans perceive physical activity?
- What can physical activity do for the average African American?
- Why is physical activity so important to the average African American?

Once these basic questions are answered from one sample of African Americans to another, then and only then can effective weight loss and weight maintenance programs work in the African American community (Desmond et al. 1990).

Conclusion

As you have surmised from this chapter's discussion, African Americans have varying perspectives about exercise, physical fitness, leisure-time physical activity, and physical activity. Regardless of all the varying opinions and perspectives, one thing is for certain—African Americans do care about their health.

I am reminded about the importance of my physical activity regimen, particularly when I was in college. In 1981, I returned to Oxford, Ohio (eight months after graduation), where I had graduated with a bachelor's degree and also played football on the varsity football team. As a former football player for Miami University (Oxford, Ohio), I arrived on campus in August 1981 completely out of shape.

In only eight months since my graduation (December 1980) and lettering in varsity football, I was not aware how much I was out of shape when I returned to campus to begin my graduate studies. In fact, many of my former teammates looked surprised when they saw me. Initially, I thought that they were surprised to see me on campus and didn't think that I was going to graduate school. However, their surprise was more due to the weight that I had gained! Eventually, one of my close friends just came out and said that I was fat!

Although it was initially a surprise to me, it really wasn't particularly if you saw my graduate student identification. I looked like a *stuffed-piglet*! Yes, little Eric "Beetle" (a nickname given to me by my football teammates) Bailey was a *stuffed-piglet*! There was no doubt about it. I had to face the facts and I did.

That's precisely when I developed a daily regimen of physical activity and a fitness work-out regimen for myself. Now that I could no longer depend on my sport of football to keep me in shape, I had to develop my own fitness regimen.

That fitness regimen involved weight-lifting and jogging. Once I completed my courses each day at the university, I headed straight to my apartment. There I lifted my weights three times a week and then I jogged around the campus—not just three days a week but every day after classes. It took me a while to get used to this fitness regimen but I did. I persisted because I knew that I couldn't continue to look like a *stuffed-piglet* anymore on campus. (Believe me, it was tough being ridiculed by my friends, particularly after being active and playing football practically all of my life.)

My fitness regimen became so much a part of my new image on campus that one of my hometown friends, Leigh Ann, who was attending Miami University, gave me my new nickname—*Daily Bailey!* Leigh Ann said she named me *Daily Bailey* simply because she would see me jogging right in her area at the same time every day. I was so precise every day that you could practically *set your watch to the precise time.*

Today, I may not have the exact same fitness regimen as I did in college, but one thing is for sure. You can call me *Daily Bailey* because I have continued a fitness regimen since then and anticipate keeping a fitness regimen for *the rest of my life!*

Postevaluation Questions

1. How can health professionals encourage more African Americans to begin an exercise and fitness regimen?

   Health professionals can encourage more African Americans to begin an exercise and physical fitness regimen by first finding out what the individual African American perceives as a regular exercise and physical fitness regimen. Then the health professional can develop an exercise and physical fitness program that incorporates their suggestions and issues of sociocultural constraints, as well as offering additional strategies for including exercise and physical fitness activities in their daily regimen.

2. What do exercise and fitness experts need to know when working with the African American community?

   When working with the African American community, exercise and physical fitness experts need to know that African Americans usually have a different perception and belief system with regard to what constitutes a healthy exercise and physical fitness regimen. Once the exercise and physical fitness experts recognize and acknowledges this slightly different orientation, then the chances of developing a culturally specific exercise and physical fitness regimen dramatically increases.

3. What can African Americans do to become more active in their exercise and fitness regimens?

   African Americans can become more active in their exercise and physical fitness regimens by first acknowledging to themselves what they perceive as a healthy exercise and physical fitness regimen. Once they recognize their own individual patterns they should compare their exercise and physical fitness strategies with several other family members and friends. Once they find other individuals who are concerned with their own exercise and physical fitness regimens, then they can begin to take small steps in implementing new exercise and physical fitness strategies.

References

Airhihenbuwa, C., Kumanyika, S., Agurs., T., and Lowe, A. 1995. Perceptions and beliefs about exercise, rest, and health among African Americans. *American Journal of Health Promotion* 9:426–429.

Babey, S., Diamant, A., Brown, R., and Hastert, T. 2005. California adolescents increasingly inactive. *UCLA Health Policy Research Brief* April:1–7.

Belza, B., Walwick, J., Shiu-Thornto, S., Schwartz, S., Taylor, M., and Lo Gerfo, J. 2004. Older adult perspectives on physical activity and exercise: Voices from multiple cultures. *Preventing Chronic Disease* 1(4):1–11.

Caspersen, C., and Merritt, R. 1992. Trends in physical activity patterns among older adults: The behavioral risk factor surveillance system, 1986–1990. *Medicine and Science in Sports and Exercise* 24 (Suppl):S26.

Centers for Disease Control and Prevention. 2004. DATA2010. Healthy People 2010 Database. Available at http://www.wonder.cdc.gov/ DATA2010.

Centers for Disease Control and Prevention. 2005. Physical activity for everyone: Physical activity terms. Available at http://www.cdc.gov/nccdphp/dnpa/physical/terms/index.htm 2005.

Centers for Disease Control and Prevention 1996. Physical activity and health: A report of the surgeon general. National Center for Chronic Disease Prevention and Health Promotion. U. S. Department of Health and Human Services.

Delany, S., Delany, A. E., and Hearth, A. H. 1994. *The Delany Sisters' Book of Everyday Wisdom*. New York: Kodansh International.

Desmond, S., Price, J., Lock, R., Smith, D., and Stewart, P. 1990. Urban black and white adolescents' physical fitness status and perceptions of exercise. *Journal of School Health* 60:220–226.

DiPietro, L., and Caspersen, C. 1991. National estimates of physical activity among white and black Americans. *Medicine and Science in Sports and Exercise* 23 (Suppl):S105.

Farmer, M., Harris, T., Madans, J., Wallace, R., Cornoni-Huntley, J., and White, L. 1989. The NHANES I epidemiologic follow-up study. *Journal of the American Geriatric Society* 37(1):9–16.

Fox, K. 1999. The influence of physical activity on mental well-being in the community. *Public Health Nutrition* 2(3A):411–418.

Giovannucci, E., Ascherio, A., Rimm, E., Colditz, G., Stampfer, M., and Willett, W. 1995. Physical activity, obesity, and risk for colon cancer and adenoma in men. *Annals of Internal Medicine* 122(5):327–334.

Gordon-Larsen, P., Griffiths, P., Bentley, M., Ward, D., Kelsey, K., Shields, K., and Ammerman, A. 2004. Barriers to physical activity: qualitative data on caregiver-daughter perceptions and practices. *American Journal of Preventive Medicine* 27(3):218–223.

Grimes, M. 2003. *Work It Out: The Black Women's Guide to Getting the Body You Always Wanted*. New York: Penguin Putnam.

Henderson, K., and Ainsworth, B. 2003. A synthesis of perceptions about physical activity among older African American and American Indian women. 93(2):313–317.

Hu, F., Stampfer, M., Colditz, G., Ascherio, A., Rexrode, K., Willett, W., Manson, J. 2000. Physical activity and risk of stroke in women. *Journal of the American Medical Association* 283(22):2961–2967.

Hu, F., Manson, J., Stampfer, M., Colditz, G., Liu, S., Solomon, C., Willett, W. 2001. Diet, lifestyle, and the risk of type 2 diabetes mellitus in women. *New England Journal of Medicine 345(11):790–797.*

Lavizzo-Mourey, R., Cox, C., Strumpf, N., Edwards, W., Lavizzo-Mourey, R., Stineman, M., and Grisso, J. A. 2001. Attitudes and beliefs about exercise among elderly African Americans in an urban community. *Journal of the National Medical Association* 93:475–480.

Nichols, D., Sanborn, C., Bonnick, S., Ben Ezra, V., Gench, B., and Di Marco, N. 1994. The effects of gymnastics training on bone mineral density. *Medicine and Science in Sports and Exercise* 26(10):1220–1225.

Nies, M., Vollman, M., and Cook, T. 1999. African American women's experience with physical activity in their daily lives. *Public Health Nursing* 16:23–31.

Paffenbarger, R., Hyde, R., Wing, A., and Steinmetz, C. 1984. A natural history of athleticism and cardiovascular health. *Journal of the American Medical Association* 252(4):491–495.

Pate, R., Pratt, M., Blair, S., Haskell, W., Macera, C., Bouchard, C., Buchner, D., Ettinger, W., Heath, G., and King, A. 1995. Physical activity and public health. A recommendation from the Centers for Disease Control and Prevention and the American College of Sports Medicine. *Journal of the American Medical Association* 273(5):402–407.

Physical Activity and Public Health. Available at http://wonder.cdc.gov/wonder/prevguid/p0000391/p0000391.asp.

Ransdell, L., and Wells, C. 1998. Physical activity in urban white, African American, and Mexican American women. *Medicine and Science in Sports and Exercise* 30:1608–1615.

Schoenborn, C. A. 1986. Health habits of U.S. adults, 1985: The Alameda 7 revisited. *Public Health Reports* 101:571–580.

Stephens, T. 1987. Secular trends in adult physical activity. *Research Quarterly in Exercise and Sports* 58:94–105.

Stephens, T., Jacobs, D., and White, C. 1985. A descriptive epidemiology of leisure-time physical activity. *Public Health Reports* 100:147–158.

Thompson, V., Baranowski, T., Cullen, K., Rittenberry, L., Baranowski, J., Taylor, W., and Nicklas, T. 2003. Influences on diet and physical activity among middle-class African American 8- to 10-year-old girls at risk of becoming obese. *Journal of the Nutrition Education and Behavior* 35: 115–123.

U.S. Department of Health and Human Services. 1996. *Physical Activity and Health: A Report of the Surgeon General.* Atlanta, GA: U.S. Department of Health and Human Services, Centers for Disease Control and Prevention, National Center for Chronic Disease and Prevention and Health Promotion.

U.S. Department of Health and Human Services. 2000. *Healthy People 2010, 2nd ed.* Washington, DC: U.S. Government Printing Office.

USA Today. 2002. Americans urged to exercise more, eat better. Available at www.usatoday.com/news/health/2002-0-05-diet-guidelines_x.htm.

USA Today. 2003. CDC tries to get Americans to exercise. Available at www.usatoday.com/news/health/2003-04-07-cdc-exercise_x.htm.

Walcott-McQuigg, J., Zerwic, J., Dan, A., and Kelley, M. 2001. An ecological approach to physical activity in African American women. *Medscape Women's Health e-Journal* 6(6).

Ward, D., Trost, S., Felton, G., Saunders, R., Parsons, M., Dowda, M., and Pate, R. 1997. Physical activity and physical fitness in African American girls with and without obesity. *Obesity Research* 5:572–577.

Weaver, R., Gaines, F., and Ebron, A. 2000. *Slim Down Sister: The African American Woman's Guide to Healthy, Permanent Weight Loss.* New York: Dutton.

White, C., Powell, K., Goelin, G., Gentry, E., and Forman, M. 1987. The behavioral risk factor surveys, IV: The descriptive epidemiology of exercise. *American Journal of Preventive Medicine* 3:304–310.

Young, D., Miller, K., Wilder, L., Yanek, L., and Becker, D. 1998. Physical activity patterns of urban African Americans. *Journal of Community Health* 23:99–112.

Young, D., Gittelsohn, J., Charleston, J., Felix-Aaron, K., and Appel, L. 2001. Motivations for exercise and weight loss among African American women: Focus group results and their contribution towards program development. *Ethnicity and Health* 6:227–245.

Adding African American Culture to Health, Physical Fitness, Diet, and Food Programs

Critical Thinking Questions

1. Why is it important to add culture to African American dietary and physical fitness regimens?
2. Is it necessary to add cultural preferences to African American dietary and physical fitness regimens?
3. What are the additional benefits to adding culture to African American dietary and physical fitness regimens?
4. Are there effective and documented culturally competent dietary and physical fitness programs for African Americans?

Introduction

Recently, there has been a lot of hype and supportive evidence of a successful diet program called the *Mediterranean-style diet* (Robertson and Smaha 2001). Researchers found evidence that subjects adhering to a Mediterranean-style diet reduced their body weight and reduced their chances of developing certain types of chronic diseases such as heart disease (Kris-Etherton et al. 2001; Singh et al. 2002). The key to this weight loss and prevention of heart disease was the introduction of the Mediterranean-style cultural pattern of eating.

Defining a Mediterranean-style diet is challenging given the broad geographical region, including at least sixteen countries, that borders the Mediterranean Sea. Nonetheless, there is a cultural dietary pattern that is characteristic of Mediterranean-style diets. This *cultural pattern* emphasizes a diet that is high in fruits, vegetables, bread, other forms of cereals, potatoes, beans, nuts, and seeds. It includes olive oil as an important fat source and dairy products, fish, and poultry consumed in low to moderate amounts; eggs consumed zero to four times weekly; and little red meat. In addition, wine is consumed in low to moderate amounts. This dietary pattern is based on food patterns typical of many regions in Greece and southern Italy in the early 1960s (Kris-Etherton et al. 2001: 1823).

The study that found supportive evidence for this Mediterranean-style diet is entitled "Effect of Weight Loss and Lifestyle Changes on Vascular Inflammatory Markers in Obese Women: A Randomized Trial." For this study, 60 women randomly assigned to the intervention group received detailed advice about how to achieve a weight reduction 10 percent or more through a low-energy Mediterranean-style diet and increased physical activity. The control group, 60 women, was given general information about healthy food choices and exercise (Esposito et al. 2003)

After two years, women in the intervention group consumed more foods rich in complex carbohydrates, monounsaturated fat, and fiber; had a lower ratio of omega-6 to omega-3 fatty acids; and had lower energy, saturated fat, and cholesterol intake than controls. Body mass index decreased more in the intervention group than in controls. In general, this study showed that a multidisciplinary program aimed to reduce body weight in obese women through lifestyle changes, including a low-energy Mediterranean-type diet and increased exercise, is feasible and gives sustained results over two years (Esposito et al. 2003: 1799).

In summary, following a *cultural dietary pattern* such as the Mediterranean-style diet can be beneficial in reducing one's body weight as well as preventing chronic diseases. In fact, the American Heart Association (AHA) Science Advisory committee reviewed the evidence supporting the benefits of a Mediterranean-style diet and stated that "it would be short-sighted to not recognize the enormous public health benefit that this diet could confer with adoption by the population-at-large if the findings are confirmed" (Kris-Etherton et al. 2001: 1825).

Defining Culture and Its Relationship to Health and Physical Fitness

Anthropology's Definition

Anthropology is a discipline unlike any other discipline in academe. Anthropology examines human populations from a holistic and comprehensive perspective. Anthropology is a study of human populations not only from a biological, physical, or genetic approach but also from a sociocultural perspective. That is, anthropologists study the everyday behavioral patterns of human cultures and how various socioeconomic or cultural factors influence our behavioral patterns. Thus, anthropology is quite distinct from other disciplines.

The four major, distinctive qualities of anthropology that set it apart from other disciplines are:

1. It's holistic;

2. It requires fieldwork;

3. It's comparative; and

4. It examines culture. (Bailey 2002: 12)

In particular, the word *culture* is used quite often to describe a wide array of human behavioral patterns. In this book, *culture* is defined as a system of shared beliefs, values, customs, and behaviors that are transmitted from generation to generation through learning.

The major attributes of culture are:

1. It's a learned process;

2. It's transmitted by symbols;

3. It adds meaning to reality;

4. It's differently shared;

5. It's integrated; and most importantly,

6. It's adaptive. (Bailey 2002: 13)

Culture relates directly to eating pattern, dieting, and fitness in the following ways. For instance, all of us learn a particular pattern of eating certain foods whether from our immediate family members or from close friends and relationships. We also learn a pattern of dieting whether from our societie's litany of diet programs or from our ethnic group. Finally, all of us learn a certain type of exercise and fitness regimen whether from our family members and/or close friends or from our social groups.

Culture is transmitted by symbols—verbally and nonverbally. In the diet and fitness field, U.S. society tends to show a preference for certain types of body types (thin to slim) in magazines, television ads, and the entertainment world as healthy, whereas those who do not fit this preference (thin to slim) are not as healthy. Symbolically, these body types (thin to slim) become the norm in society and do not allow for much variation.

Culture adds meaning to reality. In the diet and fitness field, there are thousands of experts. In this field, an individual goes through varying years of training and education to become an expert. Once the individual completes his or her training, he or she is certified with a degree or recognized in some form by society to practice or consult on diet and fitness issues. Therefore, the degree and recognition by others in society adds meaning to one's effort in becoming specialized in the diet and fitness field.

Culture is also differently shared. As discussed earlier and illustrated in a number of studies, in general, African Americans view diet, physical fitness, and body image differently than European Americans. Not only is there variation between African Americans and European Americans but there is also much variation in beliefs about diet, physical fitness, and body image *within* the African American population.

Culture is integrated. In other words, diet and physical fitness must be viewed as integrated in the totality of one's life because it is directly related to the individual's income (whether he or she can afford certain types of foods or afford joining a fitness program or not), educational level (whether he or she can comprehend certain types of diet and physical fitness regimens or not), geographic location (whether he or she lives in an area that makes diet and physical fitness accessible or not), historical issues (whether he or she has had a history, family or individual, of acknowledging the importance of diet and physical fitness or not), and political perspective (whether he or she supports diet and physical fitness programs for the general public or not).

Finally, culture is adaptive. In order for diet and physical fitness programs to be truly successful, they need to be adaptive and flexible to the needs of the consumer population thereby shifting the control of the diet and physical fitness program to the consumer as opposed to the providers (Yancey et al. 2004; Daniels et al. 2005). If this cultural strategy were incorporated more often, you would see fewer diet and physical fitness programs constantly changing in an attempt to keep up with the ever-changing consumer market.

Why Is Culture Important to Diet and Physical Fitness Programs for African Americans?

Perhaps one of the best research articles to address this question on *why is culture important to diet and physical fitness programs* is Kumanyika, Morssink, and Agurs' (1992) article entitled "Models for Dietary and

Weight Change in African American Women: Identifying Cultural Components." Their paper explored cultural factors that potentially influence the effectiveness of weight-control programs for African American women and attempted to challenge the perception that such programs operate in a culture-free context.

Kumanyika, Morssink, and Agurs (1992) stated that the absence of explicit attention to cultural aspects of behavior change as it relates to weight-control programs may result partly from the *assumption that culture is not important,* that is, from an overestimation of the level of rationality underlying individual behaviors and partly from a belief that culture is not a variable; that is, that program staff and clients are from a generally similar cultural framework and have mutual world views, definitions of self, concepts of food, and health beliefs. Yet they assert that cultural homogeneity (togetherness) cannot be assumed even among whites and far less so between African Americans and whites (Kumanyika, Morssink, and Agurs 1992: 170). Furthermore, they emphasize that even where there are similarities between African Americans and majority cultural perspectives, the assumption that African American women will perceive or respond to various messages, expectations, and situations in a manner similar to white women may be inappropriate.

For example, American culture assumes that those participating in weight-control programs are strongly motivated to be thin. Such an assumption may be a barrier in attempting to work with overweight African American women who, although they may want to weigh less and to be healthier, do not necessarily consider themselves to be unattractive or to have a weight problem and may value cosmetic aspects of body weight less as their roles change over the life span (Kumanyika, Morssink, and Agurs 1992: 172).

Another example involves the meaning of exercise. From their pilot study, Kumanyika, Morssink, and Agurs (1992) contend that black women have an orientation to exercise that was more closely tied to recreational activities or to activities that could be integrated with their other social roles versus exercise as an activity primarily geared to weight control.

In conclusion, the answer to the question on *why is culture so important to diet and physical fitness programs particularly as it relates to African American women* can be best summarized by the following quote:

> *"Efforts to make programs culturally specific to African American women may need to go beyond logistical adaptations (e.g., location or time or day when program is held) to include a behavioral analysis of weight control as it is likely to be approached by African American women within their cultural context. In other words, the way the information and related*

> *intervention tools are packaged, the assumptions and images that are expressed in the implementation of these elements, the language used to express them, and the roles of the participants can be rethought within the African American woman's cultural and social reality, that is, using African American prototypes, as defined by African Americans."*
> (Kumanyika, Morssink, and Agurs 1992: 173–174)

Adding African American Culture to Health, Physical Fitness, Diet, and Food Programs

Now that you have an appreciation for my point of view regarding the importance of culture to health and physical fitness programs and particularly its role with African American weight-loss programs, I will first define African American culture and the general cultural patterns associated with African Americans so that you can get a sense of our cultural patterns (whether you agree with them or not).

Next, I will highlight several research studies that have included African American culture into their diet, fitness, and health programs. The major purpose of highlighting these studies is to show you that it has been done successfully and that there is verifiable evidence that these programs exist (Kanders et al. 1994; Yanek et al. 2001; Walcott-McQuigg et al. 2002; McKeever et al. 2004; Paschal et al. 2004).

Third, I will highlight federal public health programs that have incorporated African American culture into their programs for the purpose of not only reaching more African Americans but also to show its effectiveness. Oftentimes, federal public health initiatives are not recognized or received well by the African American community. Well, the highlighted programs are ones that at least put a priority on recognizing certain aspects of African American culture in order to make their programs succeed.

Finally, I will highlight two books that have successfully incorporated numerous aspects of African American culture into their diet, fitness, and health programs. These books are pioneers in the field of health, diet, and physical fitness as they relate to the African American community, and they should be recognized for their efforts in making a difference.

What Is African American Culture?

Everyone has an opinion and definition of African American culture. If you ask your relatives or friends, they will have a definition that may be similar to yours or that may be completely different. Although African Americans demonstrate and express African American culture differently and similarly from one region of the United States to another or from one community to another, there are two distinctive commonalities: *shared history* and the *African American family*.

Shared history refers to a common place of origin, residence, and/or experience. Like all populations in the United States, African Americans have a shared history that is culturally based. African Americans are a people who share a common history, place of origin, language patterns, spirituality, health beliefs and values, and food preferences that engender a sense of exclusiveness and self-awareness of being a member of this ethnic group. Although African Americans may appear to be completely different from one another with regard to their physical appearance, their language patterns, their spirituality, their health beliefs and values, their interaction with one another, their socioeconomic status, and their food preferences, they all share a common history.

The African American family as a unit has a historical continuity that began not with the American experience but in Africa long before the intrusion of Europe into that continent. As early as the 1500s and 1600s, the descendants of African Americans (West Africans) were forcibly transported to South America, the Caribbean, and North America. In the process of adapting to the new environments, these West Africans merged their cultural traditions with European and Native American traditions. Although some of the cultural traditions have changed or been *Americanized*, the family unit remains constant.

The structural characteristics of the African American family today include:

1. A bilateral orientation—an equal recognition of the male and female line of descent but with an emphasis favoring the mother's kin,

2. Extended kin groups existing in a sociocultural environment in which primary-type relations are extended into the larger community,

3. Emphasis on respect for elders,

4. A high value placed on children and motherhood. (Aschenbrenner 1973; Stack 1974)

In addition to these structural characteristics, there are some other values and characteristics of African American families:

1. A high value of family and individual moral "strength" as a human quality,

2. An emphasis on family occasions and rituals,

3. Strong belief in spiritualism. (Aschenbrenner 1973; Stack 1974)

With regard to specific cultural patterns, there have been a number of generally agreed upon cultural traits associated with African

Americans. The following list is not an exclusive list, nor does it provide all the traits of African Americans; it is a baseline of cultural traits or patterns that have been associated with African Americans:

- Respect toward elders
- Reliance upon extended familial network for social, economic, and health care issues
- Strong orientation toward religious beliefs, activities, and organizations
- Outwardly expressed emotions
- Emphasis in nurturing children and participating in many rites of passages
- Preference for group activities as opposed to individual activities
- Preference for oral communication and oral history to share news and information
- Admiration of art, dance, music, and foods
- Preference for a bilateral kinship system—trace descent equally through males and females
- Preference for women and men sharing roles and responsibilities.

The African American culture list highlights the importance of culture to its people and also emphasizes how the attributes of culture relate to African American health care issues (Bailey 2002: 48–49).

Research Studies: Weight-Loss Programs Including African American Culture

Black American Lifestyle Intervention (BALI)

One project that has received a lot of attention for its incorporation of African American culture to its weight-loss program is the *Black American Lifestyle Intervention* (BALI). The BALI program is a *culturally based* weight-control program developed with the assistance of minority health professionals (Kanders et al. 1994).

In 1991, 195 obese African American women were interviewed to identify obstacles to dieting, exercise, and behavior modification, as well as attitudes and beliefs about dieting and weight loss. Information from the BALI survey was used to design the educational materials and diet that were evaluated in the pilot study.

The research team recruited African American women in Boston, Massachusetts (n = 20); New York, New York (n = 18); Houston, Texas (n = 16); and Los Angeles, California (n = 13). Women were eligible to participate if they were 40 to 64 years of age; had a body mass index (BMI) ranging from 30 to 40; earned $1,000 to $5,000 monthly; had a diastolic blood pressure (measured when the subject was not using medication) below 95 mm Hg; had a serum cholesterol below 7.76 mmol/L; and had a no history of diabetes (Kanders et al. 1994: 310).

The weight-loss phase of the pilot program lasted 10 weeks. Women were placed on a *culturally appropriate*, low-fat, nutrient-balanced, 1,200 kcal diet in which two meals were consumed as meal replacement shakes (99% lactose free). Women who were lactose intolerant were given Lactaid capsules. The shakes and Lactaid were given free of charge (Kanders et al. 1994: 311).

Participants attended one-hour group sessions led by a female African American nutritionist. The group leader distributed one-page handouts on nutrition, exercise, and behavior modification topics. Group sessions were highly interactive and included goal setting, problem solving, and role-playing. Participants received $30 at weeks 5 and 10 in exchange for completing a program evaluation form (Kanders et al. 1994: 311).

Participants were told to take three 15-minute walks per week and to increase the frequency and duration gradually until they walked 200 minutes weekly. Food and activity records were kept by the participants and were reviewed by the group leader. Additionally, all educational materials, recipes, and menu plans were reviewed by minority advisors to ensure that they were *culturally appropriate* (Kanders et al. 1994: 311).

Researchers found that of the 61 women who completed the program, participants lost an average of 3.5 percent (6.5 ± 5.3 lb) of their initial body weight in 10 weeks. Seventeen women lost 10.1 lb or more; 18 lost 5.1 lb to 10.0 lb; 14 lost 1.0 lb to 5.0 lb; 8 remained within 1 lb of baseline weight; and 4 gained weight. Most women rated the program highly and valued group support, the education component, and the BALI shakes (Kanders et al. 1994: 311).

Although the researchers state that this was only a pilot study, they emphasize strongly that the success of the BALI pilot study is attributed to the use of trained African American group leaders, ethnic foods, group support sessions, meal-replacement shakes, and a *culturally based* lifestyle education program. They further emphasize that dietitians could incorporate these features to help their minority patients achieve modest weight loss (Kanders et al. 1994: 311).

Project Joy: Faith-Based Approach

Another weight-loss program targeted for African American women that has received attention is the *Project Joy: Faith Based Cardiovascular Health Promotion for African American Women.* Project Joy was designed to address the need for well-evaluated, *culturally integrated* programs focusing on lifestyle change in African American women (Yanek et al. 2001). Participants in the pilot project named the program from a Bible verse, "... for the Joy of the Lord is your strength" (Nehemiah 8:10b). Project Joy was designed to test several strategies in the church environment to reduce cardiovascular risk in urban communities where most African American women are regular churchgoers. The overall objective was to determine the impact of active nutrition and physical activity interventions on one-year measures relating to lifestyle risk factors and cardiovascular risk profiles compared with a self-help (control) group. The study was also designed to determine the extent to which a strong spiritual component and elements of *church culture* strengthen the impact of standard behavioral group interventions in the church (Yanek et al. 2001: 69).

One church served as a pilot venue where the research team tested and refined the spiritual and *church-culture* component intervention over a 20-week period. In addition, the research team formed a Community Expert Panel to review and further refine the interventions and measurements. This group was composed of four African American churchgoing women and two African American pastors from the community. This intensive community involvement in the design of the interventions assured *cultural relevance* of the interventions and study protocols and assisted ultimately in community "ownership" of resulting programs and dissemination of results (Yanek et al. 2001: 69).

The research team divided the participants into two distinct groups: standard behavioral intervention versus spiritual intervention. Standard behavioral intervention consisted of churches holding weekly session on nutrition and physical activity in their own facilities. Each intervention session began with a weigh-in and group discussion, followed by a 30- to 45-minute nutrition education module that included a taste test or cooking demonstration. The sessions, based on a theory, were designed to enhance self-efficacy. Each session included 30 minutes of moderate-intensity aerobic activity, the nature of which varied by church; physical activities included brisk walking, water aerobics, or Tae Bo (Tae Kwan Do dance-boxing). After the first 20 weeks, lay leaders offered weekly sessions, with health educators available for support and additional information, for the remainder of the year (Yanek et al. 2001: 71). It should be noted, however, that the standard behavioral intervention sessions did include some spiritual elements primarily because participants did not believe there could be any church-based program that was not spiritual.

Spiritual intervention involved churches receiving the same sessions as the standard behavioral intervention with the addition of spiritual components and church contextual components designed by the Community Expert Panel and the research team. All weekly sessions incorporated group prayers and health messages enriched with scripture. Physical activities included aerobics to gospel music or praise and worship dance. Telephone calls from lay leaders and word of mouth from other participants motivated attendance. Church bulletins included weekly session reminders and printed messages from Project Joy, called the *Joy of Health,* on healthy eating and physical activity, accompanied by salient scriptures. The pastors offered regular information on healthy eating and physical activity from tip sheets supplied by Project Joy and distributed a monthly health newsletter, called *From the Pastor's Desk,* to the congregation. Churches also participated in at least one event per year sponsored by Project Joy, such as walk-a-thons, faith and worship dance recitals, or fruit sales, all activities that exposed other church members to the health activities of Project Joy (Yanek et al. 71–72).

Of the first 55 churches identified by the pastoral consultants and community experts, 16 churches enrolled. Of the 16 churches enrolled, 8 were Baptist (50%), 3 were independent (that is, Holiness), and 5 were externally governed (Roman Catholic, United Methodist, and AME). Four churches offered the spiritual intervention, 5 churches offered the standard intervention, and the remaining 7 churches offered self-help and included the 16 women recruited through advertising (Yanek et al. 2002: 74).

Of the 966 potential participants self-identified at the recruitment meetings, from the newsletter, or by word of mouth, 920 (95%) women were eligible. Fifty-six percent (294) of participants completed one-year follow-up biological measures and of these, 67.7 percent (199) completed all follow-up measures, including behavioral outcomes in diet and physical activity (Yanek et al. 2001: 74).

This study found that 10 percent of the participants in active church-based interventions achieved highly clinically significant improvements in cardiovascular risk profiles one year after program initiation. The research team observed significantly improved anthropometric measures, blood pressure levels, diet, and, to a lesser extent, physical activity at one year in the active intervention groups, although the magnitude of the effect was modest (Yanek et al. 2002: 76). If interventions of this nature were disseminated through large national organizations, such as the Congress of National Black Churches, for example, which represents various denominations with 65,000 churches and more than 20 million people, the public health impact could be quite considerable (Yanek et al. 2001: 80).

LEAP Weight Loss and Weight Loss Maintenance Program

Another weight-loss program that I want to mention is referred to as *LEAP*. The *Lifestyle Enhancement Awareness Program* (LEAP) examined African American women in a weight loss and weight loss maintenance program during a 32-week period (Walcott-McQuigg et al. 2002). To develop the LEAP program, qualitative and quantitative data were first gathered from 68 African American middle-income women using interviews and questionnaires. The interviews and questions were designed to identify factors in weight loss and weight loss maintenance that are both environmental (access to facilities and programs) and personal (perceptions, attitudes, stress, self-concept, and diet and exercise self-efficacy—that is, the cognitive processes in which an individual judges her ability to perform a specific behavior (i.e., a change in diet or exercise) (Walcott-McQuigg et al. 2002: 687).

The data from the study were integrated into the development of the LEAP for African American women. Therefore, LEAP incorporated African American attitudes and beliefs into the design and implementation of the program. The following research questions were examined:

- *What factors are associated with weight loss in African American women?*

- *What factors are associated with weight loss maintenance in African American women?*

The research team recruited overweight African American women from a large university medical center. To be eligible for the study, women had to be (a) a minimum of 20 percent above ideal weight for height as measured by the Metropolitan Life Insurance height–weight tables, (b) nondiabetic, (c) employed outside the home, (d) American-born, (e) willing to obtain physician approval prior to joining the program, and (f) agreeable to participating in an exercise activity three times a week for at least 20 minutes each session (Walcott-McQuigg et al. 2002: 688).

In order to participate, women signed a consent form and obtained a physician's written consent. Upon receipt of the physician's consent, women were scheduled to see a dietitian and receive preprogram assessments, which included completion of the dietary readiness questionnaire and demographics, bioelectrical impedance analysis, lipid analysis, blood pressure, and measures of the waist and hip, height and weight. An African American registered dietitian provided one hour of individualized nutrition counseling based on an evaluation of each woman's eating and activity habits. The dietitian prescribed tailored calorie-reduction diets ranging from 1400 to 1800 kilocalories a day (Walcott-McQuigg et al. 2002: 689).

The research team also provided *culturally sensitive* and relevant materials pertaining to African American women and African American culture throughout the program. The women were introduced to literature on women and body weight through interactive discussions and reading materials. These reading materials included recent articles in scientific journals and popular magazines, especially those in African American publications such as *Essence, Ebony, Heart, Body and Soul,* and *Jet.* The articles were usually personal descriptions of African American women's successful attempts at weight loss. The women were given the names and references of low-fat cookbooks, including those written for African Americans. The women also shared low-fat tasty recipes and videotapes of popular talk shows on relevant weight issues. The group viewed exercise videos and discussed them, analyzing their appropriateness for overweight and African American women (Walcott-McQuigg et al. 2002: 690).

The results of this study found that among these 23 women who completed the programs (weight loss and weight-loss maintenance), weight loss was significantly correlated with attendance and dietary readiness to decrease emotional eating. The women in the weight-loss program lost an average of 13.5 lb. The changes included reductions in body mass index, percentage body fat, waist/hip ratio, and an increase in exercise activity. The types of exercise in which the women participated during the program included walking, exercise machines at home and at health clubs, exercise videos, step aerobics, and floor exercises. As for the women in the weight loss maintenance program, they lost an average of 10.7 lb and were able to maintain a decrease in BMI and percentage body fat (Walcott-McQuigg et al. 2002: 690).

Overall, this small-scaled study was a success. Although the sample size was quite small and they relied upon convenience sampling, the research team still contends that their data shows that African American women will perform the necessary actions to lose weight if they perceive that the weight-loss program is accessible and relevant (Walcott-McQuigg et al. 2002: 693).

Wellness Within REACH (WWR)

The final weight loss and physical activity program that I want to highlight is the *Wellness Within REACH* (WWR) program in Portland, Oregon. This culturally appropriate program is designed to increase the number of African Americans leading active lifestyles, while shifting the community norm. Based out of a nonprofit organization, the African American Health Coalition (AAHC), the WWR works because the AAHC collaborates with community organizations and institutions to make a variety of activities available to community members at no cost (McKeever et al. 2004).

McKeever et al. (2004) stated that initially the AAHC had to build capacity among the African American community to facilitate the initiation of professional physical activity classes in a culturally appropriate setting. There was a gap of certified African American physical activity experts available to instruct the exercise classes. The AAHE overcame this barrier by identifying members of the African American community already in the physical activity field, who had a rapport and reputation of trust within the community, but who were not certified to teach in their respective areas of expertise (i.e., aerobics, strength training, yoga, etc.). The AAHC researched and selected a national certification program, National Endurance Sports Trainers Association (NESTA), and recruited a currently certified fitness expert to facilitate the training modules. Currently, the WWR programs include fifteen instructors, and all hold a certification for their specific form of physical activity. Additionally, there are seven individuals who are certified as Personal Trainers. Along with certifications in the specialty areas of exercise, the AAHC requires that all instructors are certified in CPR and first aid (McKeever et al. 2004: S1-95–96).

By the end of the first 10 months, WWR had developed 21 different exercise classes, and attendance data had been collected from 859 class sessions. Eight hundred eighty-seven unique community members had participated in at least one class, and most had participated several times a month. Even if a participant chose to attend a particular class only once or twice, he or she was introduced to another form of activity. In addition, the offerings span a range of physical abilities, from Senior Exercise to Kickboxing. This range helped community members remember that individuals at all levels of functioning can be physically active (McKeever et al. 2004: S1-97).

Finally, the research team stated that personal anecdotes from participants and instructors reaffirm that the program is shifting the community norm toward embracing physical activity and healthier lifestyle choices. Self-reports from numerous individuals illustrated that with the free access to, and availability of, the classes, they have been able to overcome obstacles in their lives. For example, several community members declared that they have used the opportunity to exercise to combat stress and depression due to unemployment, that they have persuaded family and friends to join them, and that they are dedicated to this "movement" that is spreading throughout the African American community. The success of the REACH Walk for Wellness, with more than 500 community members turning out for the First Annual Event, was a clear signal that people are supporting this program and that the AAHC and WWR have become household names (McKeever et al. 2004: S1-99).

Federal Programs

Usually, most of us in the community do not think that the federal government can truly develop or fund a program or a public health initiative that can have a direct positive impact in the community. All too often, federal programs sound good at press conferences and read well on paper, but to what degree these public health initiatives for the community actually improve an individual's health status is questionable, particularly as the major health disparity indicators such as heart disease, stroke, cancer, and cardiovascular disease have not improved but have increased in the African American community.

Recently, however, the Department of Health and Human Services (DHHS) announced a new initiative to improve efforts to reduce obesity among African Americans through a new partnership with national African American organizations. The National Association for Equal Opportunity in Higher Education (NAFEO; Silver Spring, Maryland) will work with the National Urban League (New York, New York), and the National Council of Negro Women (Washington, D.C.). Initiatives planned by these organizations include prevention, education, public awareness, and outreach activities intended to bring about a greater understanding of the impact of obesity on other conditions (U.S. Department of Health and Human Services 2005).

Fortunately, there are a few federal programs that have made a difference in the African American community. In fact, they are the ones that have framed their public health initiative in a *cultural* approach. Specifically, the initiatives that are mentioned use *African American cultural patterns and traditions* to not only reach the African American community but also to change some of their traditional patterns and traditions.

Heart-Healthy Home Cooking: African American Style

In 1997, the National Heart, Lung, and Blood Institute and the Office of Research on Minority Health (now known as The National Center on Minority Health and Health Disparities) at the National Institutes of Health published a booklet called *Heart-Healthy Home Cooking: African American Style.* The *Heart-Healthy Home Cooking* cookbook contains more than 20 recipes that help the individual to cut back on saturated fat, cholesterol, and sodium and still have great-tasting food. The cookbook shows individuals how to prepare their favorite African American dishes in ways that will protect them and their families from heart disease and stroke (National Institutes of Health 1997).

The *Heart-Healthy Home Cooking* cookbook is divided into three sections: Breads, Vegetables, and Side Dishes; Main Dishes; and Beverages and Desserts. Examples of some of the African American dishes are *Good-for-you Cornbread, Homestyle Biscuits, Delicious Oven French Fries,*

Candied Yams, Smothered Greens, Finger-Licking Curried Chicken, Crispy Oven-Fried Chicken, Chicken Gumbo, Spicy Southern Barbecued Chicken, Baked Pork Chops, Mock-Southern Sweet Potatoe Pie, and *1-2-3 Peach Cobbler* (National Institutes of Health 1997).

In order to make these African American dishes lower in saturated fat, cholesterol, and sodium and still have that great taste, each recipe has a special tip highlighted in the middle of the recipe. Here are a few examples:

> For Good-for-You Cornbread, the highlighted tip is "use 1% milk and a small amount of margarine to make this cornbread lower in saturated fat and cholesterol."

> For Crispy Oven-Fried Chicken, the highlighted tip is "for less fat, bake chicken in the oven instead of frying."

> For Spicy Southern Barbecued Chicken, the highlighted tip is "make barbeque sauce lower in sodium with lots of herbs and spices."

> For Baked Pork Chops, the highlighted tip is "lean cuts of fresh pork can be included in your family's heart-healthy meals."

> For Mock-Southern Sweet Potatoe Pie, the highlighted tip is "this heart-healthy pie crust is made with vegetable oil and skim milk." (National Institutes of Health 1997)

Therefore, this government funded product, *Heart-Healthy Home Cooking: African American Style*, embraced African American food preferences while also making slight changes to the *preparation* of these traditional African American dishes—a *cultural* intervention strategy that works!

Sisters Together: Move More, Eat Better Program Guide

Sister Together: Move More, Eat Better is a national initiative designed to encourage African American women 18 years of age and over to maintain a healthy weight by becoming more physically active and eating healthier foods. *Sisters Together* is an initiative of the Weight Control Information Network (WIN), a national information service of the National Institutes of Diabetes and Digestive and Kidney Diseases (NIDDK) of the National Institutes of Health (NIH). WIN, established in 1994, provides up-to-date, science-based information on obesity, physical activity, weight control, and related nutritional issues to health professionals, people who are overweight or obese, the media, Congress, and the general public (NIDDK 2003).

Sisters Together has also produced three colorful, age-appropriate, and *culturally relevant* brochures that offer African American women, their families, and their friends practical, science-based tips to help them move more, eat better, and ultimately improve their quality of life. The brochures are:

- *Celebrate the Beauty of Youth*;
- *Energize Yourself & Your Family*; and
- *Fit and Fabulous as You Mature.*

In addition to the brochures, *Sisters Together* works with national and local newspapers, magazines, radio stations, and consumer and professional organizations to further raise awareness among African American women about the health benefits of regular physical activity and healthy eating.

The *Sisters Together* initiative builds on the success of the pilot community awareness program held in Boston from 1995 to 1998. The pilot program promoted the "Move More Eat Better" message among African American women aged 18 to 35 through educational materials and planned activities such as walking groups, dance classes, and cooking demonstrations (NIDDK 2003).

To see how this initiative incorporated *African American cultural patterns and traditions* into their health promotion program, let's examine one of their brochures: *Celebrate the Beauty of Youth*. The brochure is divided into six different sections. They are:

- Why Move More and Eat Better?
- Tips on Moving;
- Look Good as You Get Fit;
- Tips on Eating Better;
- Out 'n About; and
- You Can Do it!

For example, in the section "Why Move More and Eat Better?" the brochure provides the following tips:

- Have more energy.
- Fit into hip, trendy clothes.
- Tone your body (without losing your curves!).
- Reduce stress, boredom, or the blues.
- Feel good about yourself.

For "Look Good as You Get Fit," the brochure provides these tips:

- A natural hairstyle that holds up to frequent shampoos
- A short haircut that's easy to wash and wear
- Braids, twists, or locks that stay in place while you work out
- A style that you can pull back with a headband or scrunchies

For "Tips on Eating Better," the brochure provides these tips:

- Start the day with breakfast.
- Order a hamburger without sauce or fries, or a grilled chicken sandwich (not fried).
- Choose low-fat or nonfat milk instead of whole milk or a regular milkshake.
- Eat more fruits, vegetables, and whole grains.
- Go easy on mayonnaise, creamy sauces, and added butter.
- Don't let soda or other sweets crowd out healthy foods.
- Drink eight 8-ounce glasses of water every day. (NIDDK 2003)

Unlike the previous federal government initiative, this program developed age-appropriate and culturally relevant brochures to reach the young, middle-age, and mature markets of the African American women population—a *cultural* intervention strategy that also works!

Fruits and Vegetables: Men Eat 9 a Day

The *Fruits and Vegetables: Men Eat 9 a Day* initiative is an outgrowth of the National Cancer Institute's (NCI) 5 A Day Program. The 5 A Day Program is a national program that approaches Americans with a simple, positive message: Eat 5 or more servings of vegetables and fruit daily for better health. The consumption of 5 or more servings of vegetables and fruit daily for better health was supported by a diverse and convincing body of evidence. Further evidence has accumulated to support the hypothesis that a diet rich in vegetables and fruit reduces the risk of cancer and other chronic diseases. Research also shows that people with higher fruit and vegetable intakes tend to eat fewer calories overall and have better weight control (Campbell et al. 1999).

The *Fruits and Vegetables: Men Eat 9 a Day* initiative, however, is directed to all men especially African American men. The marketing of this new initiative includes a national Web site (http://5aday.gov/9aday/black-menshealth/diet/diet.html) and colorful brochures showing African American men promoting fruit and vegetable consumption and a nine-step approach to eating healthier.

The nine-step approach is as follows:

- Have a glass of 100 percent juice in the morning.
- Snack on fresh fruit throughout the day. Grab an apple or banana on your way out the door.
- Eat a big salad at lunch.
- Snack on raw veggies.
- Keep dried fruit in your desk drawer for a quick snack.
- Enjoy your favorite beans and peas. For extra flavor, use lean ham instead of bacon.
- Eat your greens—just watch the fat. Use lean meats for flavor instead of ham hocks and fatback.
- Eat at least two vegetables with dinner.
- Eat fruit for desert. (National Cancer Institute 2003)

Whether this cultural health intervention campaign is a success or not only time will tell. It is encouraging to see the effort is there and at least they have incorporated a number of African American symbols and traditional food staples in a cultural intervention approach.

Books

Before I conclude this chapter, I want to recognize two books that have successfully incorporated numerous aspects of *African American culture* into their diet, fitness, and health programs. These books are pioneers in the field of health, diet, and fitness as they relate to the African American community and should be recognized for their ground-breaking efforts. These books are entitled *Good Health for African Americans* by Barbara M. Dixon and *Slim Down Sister* by Roniece Weaver, Fabiola Gaines, and Angela Ebron.

In her book *Good Health for African Americans,* Dixon (1994) stated that it was her desire to create an effective nutritional and lifestyle self-help program specifically for African Americans. The book examined African Americans' old traditions that influence the foods we choose, modern eating habits, destructive lifestyle practices, black stress, and genetic factors.

The nutritional program that Barbara Dixon developed was called the *Sankofa program*. Sankofa, which is an African proverb meaning "learning from the past, building the future," is a program that is a self-help nutrition and lifestyle plan. It is grounded in what is best about our African American past and all the healthful nutritional practices that are compatible with our *culture*. It also incorporates all the modern knowledge about the effects of nutrition on African American health (Dixon 1994: 111).

The *Sankofa program* is based upon Dixon's (1994) five guiding principles:

- Variety is the key to good nutrition.
- Plan gradual change not instant makeovers.
- Add foods that help you fight diseases.
- Set sensible goals and stay flexible.
- Keep things simple, and introduce small changes one at a time. (Dixon 1994: 112)

Overall, Dixon's (1994) book was well-received by the African American community and in particular it helped to open up new areas of cultural health intervention with regard to dietary pattern as it relates to African Americans.

The next book is *Slim Down Sister*—the first weight-loss book written especially for African American women. This book addresses the serious health concerns facing African American women today and offers a comprehensive, get-down-to-it program of diet and exercise that empowers sisters to take control of their weight and health.

In their book *Slim Down Sister,* Weaver, Gaines, and Ebron (2000) offer insight into why weight loss is more difficult for African American women and they pull no punches. They state:

> *"We're honest about the facets of our lifestyle that keep us from our weight-loss goals. We'll key you in to the special health risks associated with overweight that black women face, and help you understand how resolving to get fit is the first step to prolonging your life. We'll show you how to take the best parts of sisterhood—like our positive self-image—and make them work for you, not against you."* (Weaver, Gaines, and Ebron 2000: 4)

In addition, the book includes an exercise program designed by a sister certified fitness trainer that's especially for African American women. In general, *Slim Down Sister* continues to be a highly effective health, fitness, and weight-loss book designed especially for African American women.

Conclusion

All too often, we hear or read about from other scholars, researchers, and/or published articles that there is no good evidence on how *culture* can be added to health, physical fitness, diet, and food programs for African Americans. Well, in this chapter, I provided you an abundance of evidence from the latest research studies, federal programs, and books that have all incorporated various aspects of African American culture into their specific health, fitness, diet, and food programs. Not only have these programs incorporated various aspects of African American culture, but these programs also show that they have been successful in using these African American cultural patterns, beliefs, and values within their particular programs. Along the same lines then, the next and final chapter of this book will introduce my *New Black Cultural Diet*™ plan.

Postevaluation Questions

1. How can health professionals learn to incorporate more culturally competent strategies into their diet and fitness regimens for African Americans?

    Health professionals can incorporate more culturally competent strategies into their diet and physical fitness regimen for African Americans by spending more time observing how African Americans exercise and by spending more time asking specific questions about what individual African Americans would prefer in their diet and physical fitness regimens.

2. Do most African Americans prefer more of a culturally competent approach to their diet and fitness regimens?

    In general, a majority of African Americans do prefer more of a culturally competent approach to their diet and physical fitness regimens. Depending on the individual orientation of the African American and other factors, such as socioeconomic status, educational level, and region of the country, most African Americans prefer familiarity in their exercise and physical fitness regimens.

3. What can African Americans do to make an exercise and dietary regimens easier to incorporate into their lifestyle?

    African Americans can make their exercise and dietary regimens a part of their lifestyle simply by establishing health and physical fitness as a high priority in their lives. It is important to include additional exercise and physical fitness strategies in small increments throughout one's daily and weekly lifestyle so that the individual

African American can see how a regular regimen of exercise and physical fitness can fit into anyone's busy lifestyle.

References

Aschenbrenner, J. 1973. Extended families among black Americans. *Journal of Comparative Family Studies* 4:257–268.

Bailey, E. 2002. *Medical Anthropology and African American Health.* Westport, CT: Bergin & Garvey.

Campbell, M., Dmark-Wahnefried, W., Symons, M., Kalsbeek, W., Doods, J., Cowan, A., Jackson, B., Motsinger, B., Hoben, K., Lashley, J., Demissie, S., and McClelland, J. 1999. Fruit and vegetable consumption and prevention of cancer: The black churches united for better health project. *American Journal of Public Health* 89:1390–1396.

Daniels, S, Arnett, D., Eckel, R., Gidding, S., Hayman, L., Kumanyika, S., Robinson, T., Scott, B., Jeor, S., and Williams, C. 2005. Overweight in children and adolescents: Pathophysiology, consequences, prevention, and treatment. *Circulation* 111:1999–2012.

Dixon, B. 1994. *Good Health for African Americans.* New York: Crown Publishers.

Esposito, K., Pontillo, A., Di Palo, C., Giugliano, G., Masella, M., Marfella, R., and Giugliano, D. 2003. Effect of weight loss and lifestyle changes on vascular inflammatory markers in obese women: A randomized trial. *Journal of the American Medical Association* 289:1799–1804.

Kanders, B., Ullman-Joy, P., Foreyt, J., Heymsfield, S., Heber, D., Elashoff, R., Ashley, J., Reeves, R., and Blackburn, G. 1994. The Black American Lifestyle Intervention (BALI): The design of a weight loss program for working-class African American women. *Journal of the American Dietetic Association* 94:310–312.

Kris-Etherton, P., Eckle, R., Howard, B., St. Jeor, S., and Bazzarre, T. 2001. Lyon diet program/American Heart Association Step I dietary pattern on cardiovascular disease. *Circulation* 103:1823–1825.

Kumanyika, S., Morssink, C., and Agurs, T. 1992. Models for dietary and weight change in African American women: Identifying cultural components. *Ethnicity and Disease* 2:166–175.

McKeever, C., Faddis, C., Koroloff, N., and Henn, J. 2004. Wellness within REACH: Mind, body, and soul: A no-cost physical activity program for African Americans in Portland, Oregon to combat cardiovascular disease. *Ethnicity and Disease* 14(summer):S1-93–S1-101.

National Cancer Institute. 2003. *Fruits and Vegetables: Men Eat 9 a Day.* Washington, DC: NIH Publication 03-5332. Available at http://5aday.gov/9aday/blackmenshealth/diet/diet.html.

National Institutes of Health. 1997. *Heart Healthy Home Cooking: African American Style.* Washington, DC: NIH Publication 97-3792.

NIDDK (National Institutes of Diabetes and Digestive and Kidney Disorders). 2003. *Sisters Together: Move More, Eat Better Program.* Available at www.niddk.nih.gov.

Paschal, A, Lewis, R., Martin, A., Dennis-Shipp, D., and Simpson, D. 2004. Baseline assessment of the health status and health behaviors of African Americans participating in the activities for life program: A community-based health intervention program. *Journal of Community Health* 29(4):305–318.

Robertson, R., and Smaha, J. 2001. Can a Mediterranean-style diet reduce heart disease? *Circulation* 103:1821–1822.

Singh, R., Dubnov, G., Niaz, M., Ghosh, S., Sing, R., Rastogi, S., Manor, O., Pella, D., and Berry, E. 2002. Effect of an Indo-Mediterranean diet on progression of coronary artery disease in high risk patients (Indo-Mediterranean Diet Heart Study): A randomised single-blind trial. *Lancet* 360:1455–1461.

Stack, C. 1974. *All Our Kin: Strategies for Survival in a Black Community.* New York: Harper & Row.

U.S. Department of Health and Human Services. 2005. HHS launches African American obesity initiative. U.S. DHHS. Office of Minority Health Press Release. Available at http://www.os.dhhs.gov/news/press/2005pres/20050407.html.

Walcott-McQuigg, J., Chen, S.-P., Davis, K., Stevenson, E., Choi, A., and Suparat, W. 2002. Weight loss and weight loss maintenance in African American women. *Journal of the National Medical Association* 94:686–694.

Weaver, R., Gaines, F., and Ebron, A. 2000. *Slim Down Sister: The African American Woman's Guide to Healthy Weight Loss.* New York: Dutton.

Yancey, A., Kumanyika, S., Ponce, N., McCarthy, W., Fielding, J., Leslie, J., and Akbar, J. 2004. Population-based interventions engaging communities of color healthy eating and active living: A review. *Preventing Chronic Disease: Public Health Research, Practice, and Policy* 1(1):1–24.

Yanek, L., Becker, D., Moy, T., Gittelsohn, J., and Koffman, D. 2001. Project joy: Faith based cardiovascular health promotion for African American women. *Public Health Reports* 116 (Suppl 1):68–81.

PART III
THE NEW CULTURAL APPROACH

This section introduces the author's New Black Cultural Diet™. This new cultural approach to weight loss will allow the reader to investigate key cultural health and fitness issues that may be preventing the individual African American from overcoming these cultural barriers that are related to good health and physical fitness.

THE NEW BLACK CULTURAL DIET AND LIFESTYLE

Critical Thinking Questions

1. Is there a need to develop a new dietary plan for African Americans?
2. Why is it difficult to design a dietary plan for African Americans?
3. How can African American cultural traits be added to a dietary plan?
4. Is there a distinction between general health issues and cultural health issues associated with African Americans?

Introduction

So here we are—the final chapter of this book. It is the most important chapter because I will share with you my formula, strategy, better yet my *culturalized* health, diet, and physical fitness approach for optimal health and weight maintenance specifically designed for the African American population. I think one of the most effective strategies in solving practical health care issues such as overweight and obesity in the African American community is for us to begin to understand not only how the community perceives (values, beliefs, and attitudes) the health issue but also how to develop interventions from the community's "cultural" base of orientation (perspective) to the issues of overweight, obesity, health, and fitness. That is why the New Black Cultural Diet is based on a "cultural framework or model."

The New Black Cultural Diet and Lifestyle: The Model

Definitions and Terminology

As stated earlier in this book, there will be no special diet regimen that you will have to follow; there will be no particular foods that you have to avoid; and there will be no particular exercises that you have to do! The only thing that you really have to do is to be truthful, direct, and *real* with yourself in finding out, or better yet *self-diagnosing* yourself, regarding what are the reasons causing you to gain weight or what are the reasons that can help you lose and maintain that weight loss.

My unique approach to the health, diet, and fitness issues associated with African Americans involves using the traits and patterns associated with "our culture" to help us in overcoming our overweight and obesity problems. What does this mean? It means that the only requirement of this New Black Cultural Diet plan is to ask yourself or to ask the person who is attempting to lose weight some key "cultural health and physical fitness questions." The key "cultural health and physical fitness questions" are based on the concept referred to as "cultural appropriateness."

Cultural appropriateness means developing a system of shared beliefs, values, traditions, and patterns that meet the cultural standards of the individual and/or group (Bailey 1994; 2000). Prevention interventions need to become more *culturally appropriate* by taking into consideration ethnic group differences in social, psychological, environmental, and cultural aspects of health (Robinson and Killen 2001). Jacobson et al. (2002) state specifically that weight-control initiatives, if *culturally adapted*, may show considerably more promise and more favorable outcomes that non–culturally adapted weight-control initiatives. This has particular relevance for obesity prevention interventions, as African American boys, girls, women, and men represent groups at highest risk and there are known cultural differences that may affect intervention design and implementation.

The term "cultural appropriateness" is used instead of "cultural competence" simply because most individuals and, particularly, groups have a much more difficult time in *truly understanding and embracing* the values, beliefs, attitudes, traditions, and patterns of another individual and/or group. The fact that all of us, including myself, have certain perspectives and values that we adhere to and that we follow on a day-to-day basis is normal. The fact that I may have a different set of values, beliefs, and patterns associated with health, fitness, and diet from my mother, brothers, cousins, and even my wife is normal. Yet, when we are asked to *truly understand and embrace* another person's or group's value system and traditions, we often have a difficult time in accomplishing this task. That is why I chose the term "cultural appropriateness." I am attempting to develop an obesity intervention program (health, fitness, and diet program) that meets the *cultural standards* (values, beliefs, traditions, and patterns) of several different cultural groups in the African American community (*men, women, boys, and girls*). Thus, the New Black Cultural Diet program is based on the cultural values, traditions, and patterns of African Americans in the United States.

Culturally Appropriate Health Intervention Strategies for Specific Segments of the African American Population

The following paragraphs highlight selected culturally appropriate (cultural relativistic) research studies that strongly suggest the importance of recognizing culture in the model of health intervention for specific segments of the African American population. Four specific segments of the African American population are highlighted.

Culture and African American Elderly

African American elders are a diverse group, and it is important to recognize this group's heterogeneity (Brangman 1995). No typical African American elder exists. They can vary from an elder living in the rural South to an elder in an urban area in the Northeast (Brangman 1995). Brangman states that they may have been born in the northern or southern parts of the United States or be members of a subgroup, as are immigrants from various parts of the Caribbean, such as Jamaica or Haiti. Their history, religious, educational, socioeconomic, and marital statuses and cultural backgrounds must be taken as a starting point for understanding the individual while avoiding overgeneralizations and stereotypes (Brangman 1995: 16; Mouton, Johnson, and Cole 1995).

Martin and Panicucci's (1996) study of 40 elderly African American women's health behaviors and beliefs highlighted the difference in this study's results versus stereotypical beliefs associated with elderly African American women. Findings revealed that Southern, community-living African American older women generally have a high level of adherence to commonly recommended health promotion/disease prevention habits.

Martin and Panicucci stipulated that a most likely explanation for the high levels of adherence may stem from their cultural and religious doctrines that discourage certain unhealthy practices such as excessive alcohol consumption, cigarette smoking, and ineffective coping outlets. Because study findings indicate that African American older women want to maintain their health, increased attention must be directed to the importance of primary prevention behaviors as an assertion of control over one's future health, well-being, and quality of life (Martin and Panicucci 1996: 17; Bailey 2000).

Culture and African American Women

In recent years, there has been a new consciousness and awareness concerning women's health within the biomedical and health care community (Pinn 1996). In 1990, the National Institutes of Health (NIH) established the Office of Research on Women's Health for the purpose of strengthening and developing research initiatives for women in all communities. In fact, one of NIH's specific initiatives in 1995 focused on behavioral and cultural factors related to women and disease prevention/intervention (Pinn 1996: 10).

One particular large-scale study that has developed from this research initiative on women's health is the Black Women's Health Study. Funded by the National Cancer Institute and conducted by a team of epidemiologists from Boston and Howard Universities, the Black Women's Health Study is the largest epidemiological study of African American women yet conducted (Rosenberg, Adams-Campbell, and Palmer 1995). This study expects to find answers concerning issues of obesity and diseases; relation of physical activity to cardiovascular disease, diabetes mellitus, and breast cancer; and the relation of cigarette smoking to cardiovascular disease (Rosenberg, Adams-Campbell, and Palmer 1995). Moreover, the answers to these health issues will provide some general insight into the cultural health beliefs associated with physical fitness, exercise, and health seeking patterns among African American women.

Yet there still remains a gap of information concerning how culture influences health practices among African American women (Mouton et al. 1997). Kathleen Jennings (1996), a nurse practitioner, highlighted six cultural relativistic (appropriate) intervention strategies that nurse practitioners should use when working with African American women. They are described as follows:

1.   Appreciate: relating sister to sister.

2.   Negotiate: creating community kinship.

3.   Integrate: combining health beliefs and health behaviors.

4.   Educate: empowering women through knowledge.

5.   Advocate: "I've got your back" (explained later).

6.   EVALUATE: application of the nursing process. (Jennings 1996: 57)

For example, relating sister to sister implies that the nurse practitioner must develop "sister circles" within African American communities for the purpose of influencing cancer health behaviors. In order to develop these "sister circles," Jennings suggests that nurse practitioners must: (1) develop an understanding of the African American culture, its issues, its values, and its health concerns; (2) seek out the formal sister circles in the community; (3) be visible in places where women meet; and (4) identify and respect the reverent power of community leaders.

Second, Jennings suggests that empowering women through knowledge means the following:

1. Screening programs should be designed to give accurate information, not just provide an examination.

2. Educational programs should address the psychosocial issues of being black and female.

3. Educational programs should be user-friendly.

4. Educational programs should provide information regarding community resources available for clients to access. These types of educational strategies will truly empower women with the knowledge to change health behaviors.

Finally, Jennings suggests that "I've got your back," referring to being committed to support someone in need, is an important concept in the African American community. Nurse practitioners must be committed in the fight against cancer in order to win the trust of the community and to create a perception of a caring attitude (Jennings 1996: 57).

In summary, although the health care field has awakened to the specific health issues concerning African American women, there still remains a lack of information and understanding about how cultural factors influence health behavior. The use of small focus group sessions with African American women will provide answers to a number of health issues affecting African American women's health. A cultural relativistic perspective as it relates to African American women's health is desperately needed.

Culture and African American Men

Year after year, the health data associated with African American men continue to show a strikingly large disparity among health outcomes when compared with other segments of the U.S. population. In comparison with life expectancy, African American men continue to have the lowest life expectancy (68 years) among racial groups in the United States.

As for research on the relationship between culture and health care practices among African American men, very little research has been conducted and even the research that has been conducted has been very minimal or very generalized (American Institute for Cancer Research 1997; U.S. Department of Health and Human Services 1997). One particular study interested in the African American adult males' knowledge and perceptions of prostate cancer found that cultural health beliefs influenced health care seeking (Price et al. 1993). The results from 290 randomly selected African American men living in the seven largest cities in Ohio (Columbus, Cincinnati, Cleveland, Toledo, Dayton, Akron, and Canton) revealed that a majority of men did not perceive themselves as susceptible to prostate cancer. Additionally, 45 percent of the men perceived prostate cancer as a death sentence, and another 28 percent were not sure if it would kill them (Price et al. 1993: 945). Price and colleagues stated that when you add to this perception the fact that one in five men claimed that the cost of a prostate examination would be a significant barrier to having their prostates examined, you have a condition that helps explain why so many African American males have prostate cancer diagnosed at advanced stages.

With regard to prostate cancer intervention, Price and colleagues suggest that health educators must realize that unless they oversell the importance of their interventions, they may create a problem of "victim blaming." In other words, some health educators may believe that African American males do not engage in preventive behaviors only because they are ignorant of their risks and the signs and symptoms of prostate cancer (Price et al. 1993: 946). Price and colleagues contend that not only does this type of thinking fail to appreciate how health behaviors develop and are sustained, but also a major portion of the higher prostate cancer mortality rate in African American males is related to socioeconomic inequalities and discrimination and its relation to lack of access to health care.

In conclusion, Price et al. (1993) suggest that there is a need for increased public education directed specifically at African American males. Cultural relativistic (appropriate) education intervention should be directed toward symptom recognition and more realistic assessments of the benefits of regular prostate cancer examinations (Price et al. 1993: 947). Moreover, clinicians who have direct cultural experiences with African American men can help focus specific education interventions and research efforts that provide relevant information to develop appropriate prostate cancer initiatives for specific populations of African American men (Guidry, J., Mathews-Juarez, P., Copeland, V. 2003; Weinrich et al. 1998).

Culture and African American Adolescent Females

To determine whether obesity prevention programs could work effectively in the African American community, Stolley and Fitzgibbon (1997) designed a culturally specific (appropriate) obesity prevention for low-income, African American adolescent females and their mothers who live in Chicago's inner city. Using the information gathered in a pilot project, Stolley and Fitzgibbon developed a curriculum that addressed the particular cultural and social needs of this population.

First, Stolley and Fitzgibbon felt that parental participation with this population was imperative given the mothers' limited access to dietary and physical activity information, their need for nutrition and health knowledge, and their need for support in making dietary changes. Second, the program was held at a local tutoring program. Third, all activities involving tasting foods, comparing high-fat to low-fat foods, changing recipes, and planning meals were done with foods identified in 24-hour recalls gathered in the pilot project. In addition, subjects in this program were asked to bring in their favorite recipes of foods to be analyzed for fat and caloric content. Fourth, attention to the availability of certain products was given in classes addressing menu planning. Fifth, culturally relevant music and dance were used for a number of exercise and diet-related activities. Finally, appropriate materials gathered from magazines geared toward African Americans were distributed and reviewed for important information on diet and exercise (Stolley and Fitzgibbon 1997: 155).

Stolley and Fitzgibbon found that over the course of a twelve-week program treatment, mothers exhibited a significant decrease in saturated fat and dietary fat, coupled with an increase in parental support. After the intervention, the mothers who participated in the program reported receiving less than 32 percent of their calories from fat and an average intake of 11.5 grams of saturated fat, compared with a pretreatment diet of 40 percent daily calories from fat and nearly 14 grams of saturated fat (Stolley and Fitzgibbon 1997: 159). Stolley and Fitzgibbon stated that the interventions had a positive effect on mothers' levels of support and role modeling of healthy eating behavior for their daughters.

The treatment daughters reported only minor changes in their percentage of calories from fat at post-treatment. Although daughters' behaviors changed only minimally during the twelve-week intervention, Stolley and Fitzgibbon contend that the mothers' modeling behaviors will change the daughters' behaviors in time. Follow-up data will offer insight regarding this issue (Stolley and Fitzgibbon 1997: 159).

Along with parental participation, Stolley and Fitzgibbon believed that other components were imperative to the success of the program. These cultural relativisitic components included:

1. Conducting the program in a safe and familiar community location;

2. Incorporation of culturally appropriate music, dance, and media;

3. Acknowledgment and knowledge of neighborhood markets in which families shop;

4. Acknowledgment and inclusion of foods commonly prepared and eaten by families as identified through 24-hour recalls;

5. Attention to the challenges of adopting a low-fat dietary plan within a strict financial budget. (Stolley and Fitzgibbon 1997:163)

Other factors that Stolley and Fitzgibbon (1997) believe could enhance the effectiveness of the program include: (1) a longer-term intervention, (2) follow-up booster sessions to support maintenance of dietary changes, (3) inclusion of a more intensive exercise component, and (4) spending class time on actual preparation of low-fat meals.

In conclusion, this obesity prevention program for African American adolescent females attempted not only to work within the social and cultural parameters of this particular African American population but also to challenge many of the cultural dietary eating patterns of African American adolescent females and their mothers (Walcott-McQuigg et al.). This cultural relativistic approach to dietary intervention and weight control for African American adolescent females provides a framework for understanding how cultural and social factors influence positive health behavioral patterns.

Categories of Cultural Appropriateness Components

In order to evaluate, diagnose, and ask the key *cultural health and physical fitness questions* to yourself or another person, we must divide the *cultural appropriateness* components into two components. They are *surface structure* and *deep structure* (Robinson and Killen 2001). Although our major objective is to better understand the *deep structural* cultural components as to why we may have a weight problem, the New Black Cultural Diet and Lifestyle will also help us to evaluate the *surface structural* cultural components as to how we can make the new diet and fitness program more appealing to our cultural preferences.

Surface structural cultural components refer to culturally matched elements that are similar to your cultural preferences. For example, in deciding upon a weight-loss program, an African American may have a preference to join a weight-loss program that has foods that match his or her cultural food preferences; that has facilitators who are of similar ethnicity; that has facilitators who are of similar socioeconomic status; that has facilitators who are of similar religious and spiritual denomination; that describes the weight-loss program in a manner that he or she is accustomed to; that uses specific colors and symbols that he or she is accustomed to; and that has an exercise regimen similar to his or her health fitness pattern.

Perhaps another way to explain the *surface structural* cultural components is as follows:

- Eating similar traditional African American soul food, but prepared without the extra sauces, sodium, and fat

- Having an African American instructor for the weight-loss program

- Having the instructor of the weight-loss program similar in age and socioeconomic standing
- Having the instructor of the weight-loss program from the same religious denomination
- Having the instructional materials easy to read and understand
- Having the instructional materials presented in colors and symbols associated with African American culture
- Having exercises that are easy to accomplish.

Deep structural cultural components refer to culturally matched elements that are similar to one's cultural values, beliefs, attitudes, and social and historical orientation. For example, in deciding upon a weight-loss program, an African American may prefer to join a weight-loss program that takes into account African American cultural traits and patterns such as importance of family, present orientation, importance of religiosity, sense of historical racism and prejudice, and use of social support as a coping element (Robinson and Killen 2001: 275).

In other words, another way to explain the *deep structural* cultural components is as follows:

- Allowing close family members and extended family members to share their opinions and perspectives about overweight, obesity, fitness, and food preferences
- Focusing on the reasons you have a weight problem and how you are going to immediately benefit (physically, socially, emotionally, and economically) from losing and maintaining the weight loss as opposed to the benefits in the future
- Having an instructor or other members of the weight-loss program who have similar religious and spiritual beliefs associated with health and fitness
- Having the instructor show respect and not talk down or demean you
- Using and socializing with support groups that not only share similar health and fitness beliefs and practices but also will motivate and encourage you to stay on the weight-loss program.

In general, the *surface structural* and *deep structural* cultural appropriateness components are designed not only to get you and/or the instructor of the weight-loss program in recognizing your cultural health and fitness preferences but also to get you and/or the instructor to find out the *real reasons* why you are having a weight problem.

Cultural Health and Physical Fitness Questions

Introduction

Now that we have defined the difference between the two concepts—*surface structural* and *deep structural* cultural appropriateness components—and showed how both concepts play a vital part in highlighting your cultural health and fitness preferences, as well as finding out the real reasons why you are having a weight problem, we are ready to prepare the critical *cultural health* and *physical fitness questions*. These questions center around the four key elements to health and fitness: *body image, food selection, food preparation, and exercise.*

These four key elements to health and fitness are the focus of this book and the foundation of my New Black Cultural Diet and Lifestyle. After researching a number of diet plans, a number of new diet books (trendy and most-advertised), a number of research journal articles, and listening to a number of health, fitness, and diet experts, I felt that these four key elements to health and physical fitness (*body image, food selection, food preparation, and exercise*) provide the basis on which to challenge and change the cultural preferences among African Americans regarding foods, dieting, and fitness. If *culturally approached* in a *culturally-appropriate strategy*, then we really can get to the *real reasons* why so many African Americans are having problems with their weight, thereby *reducing* the number of African Americans who are overweight and obese in the United States.

One way to ask the questions and to challenge these cultural preferences is to use the six attributes of culture to construct the *cultural health and physical fitness questions*. The six major attributes of culture are:

- Culture is learned;
- Culture is transmitted by symbols;
- Culture is integrated into your total lifestyle;
- Culture adds meaning to reality;
- Culture is differently shared; and
- Culture is adaptive.

From these *six cultural attributes* derive the *set of six cultural health and physical fitness questions*. To reiterate, the major purpose of these types of questions and the cultural approach being used is primarily to get you to feel at ease and culturally comfortable to uncover the real reasons why you may be having a problem with your weight and to constructively do something about it. Let's see how it works.

Body Image

According to psychologists, *body image* is the internal, subjective representation of physical appearance and bodily experience, whereas *body type* preference is the ideal against which one measures or compares one's own body's size and shape (Thompson and Smolak 2001). In other words, body image is your perception of how your body looks, and body type is how your body compares with other body types. These two concepts—body image and body type preference—are very important factors as to why African Americans have this (what I refer to as) "flexible cultural definition of healthiness."

The *cultural health and physical fitness questions* to ask yourself are as follows:

1. Culture is learned.
   - *How did I learn my preferred body image?*
   - *How am I going to change my body type to the body image that I prefer?*

2. Culture is transmitted by symbols.
   - *How will my body look when it is larger?*
   - *How will my body look when it is leaner?*

3. Culture is integrated in your total lifestyle.
   - *How will my larger body size affect my quality of life (economically, physically, spiritually, socially, and mentally)—day to day?*
   - *How will my leaner body size improve my quality of life (economically, physically, spiritually, socially, and mentally)—day to day?*

4. Culture adds meaning to reality.
   - *How have I mentally accepted that my larger size will most likely influence other family members and friends to be larger also?*
   - *How will my leaner body size influence other family members and friends?*

5. Culture is differently shared.
   - *How is my larger body size different from other family members or friends?*

- *How will my leaner body size be different from other family members and friends?*

6. Culture is adaptive.

    - *How will my larger body size change who I am?*
    - *How will my leaner body size change who I am?*

Interestingly, answers to this set of six *cultural health and physical fitness questions* will help you to re-assess your body image and body type as it is now and how it may be in the future. When faced with such revealing images and the impact that your body size will have on others, you will most likely take constructive steps in challenging and changing your body image.

Food Selection

According to *Webster's Dictionary*, *food* is defined as any substance that provides the nutrients necessary to maintain life and growth when ingested. When food is ingested and consumed in a regular pattern, we are referring to *food habits* (Kittler and Suchler 2000; 2).

Like all groups of people, African Americans have established certain types of traditional food habits. *Soul food* is one term often used to describe African Americans' traditional food habits. However, African Americans consume a much wider diversity of foods than the stereotypical soul food diet. Depending on the region of the country, proximity to other cultural groups, assimilation with mainstream lifestyles, and individual preferences, African American food selection may be as diverse as any other group.

The *cultural health and physical fitness questions* that you may ask yourself are as follows:

1. Culture is learned.

    - *How did I learn my preferences for certain types of foods?*
    - *How am I going to change the selection of foods that I know are not healthy for me?*

2. Culture is transmitted by symbols.

    - *How am I perceived by other family members and friends when I purchase unhealthy foods on a regular basis?*
    - *How am I perceived by other family members and friends when I purchase healthier foods on a regular basis?*

3.   Culture is integrated into your total lifestyle.

- *How will the unhealthy foods that I consume affect my quality of life (economically, physically, spiritually, socially, and mentally)—day to day?*

- *How will the healthy food selections improve my quality of life (economically, physically, spiritually, socially, and mentally)—day to day?*

4.   Culture adds meaning to reality.

- *How do the unhealthy foods that I consume daily affect my mental well-being?*

- *How will the healthy food selections affect my mental well-being?*

5.   Culture is differently shared.

- *How are my unhealthy food selections different and/or similar to other family members and friends?*

- *How are my healthy food selections different and/or similar to other family members and friends?*

6.   Culture is adaptive.

- *How are my unhealthy food selections affecting who I am?*

- *How are my healthy food selections affecting who I am?*

Your answers to this set of six cultural health and physical fitness questions will help you to not only recognize how you learned your individual food preferences (parents and extended family food pattern) but, most importantly how your unhealthy food selections are caused or highly influenced by your immediate social and familial environment. When faced with the reality that your preferred food selections are causing you more and more health problems (bloating, breathing difficulty, and high blood pressure), you will most likely take constructive steps in challenging and changing your food selections to foods that truly benefit you nutritiously while also tasting good.

Nonetheless, perhaps the biggest change in your diet may come from the selection and daily consumption of water. According to Dr. Walter Willett of the Harvard School of Public Health:

"For plain old topping off your tank, water is hard to beat. It has 100 percent of what you need—pure H2O—and no calories or additives." (Willett 2001)

Food Preparation

Earlier in this book, Whitehead (1992) reminded us that *soul food* is more than just the type of specific foods associated with Africans and African Americans but also involves the *preparation styles* of these foods. Whether it is cooking foods in a slow stewing manner, or frying, or even spicing up foods with sugar, salt, or peppers, *soul food* is a special taste and flavor with foods that have a lot of history.

The *cultural health and physical fitness questions* that you may ask yourself are as follows:

1.   Culture is learned.

   • *How did I learn how to prepare my foods?*

   • *How I am going to prepare my foods healthier?*

2.   Culture is transmitted by symbols.

   • *How am I perceived by other family members and friends when I always fry or add the extra sugar, salt, peppers, and other flavorings to my food?*

   • *How am I perceived by other family members and friends when I always reduce or avoid adding extra sugar, salt, peppers, and other flavorings to my food?*

3.   Culture is integrated in your total lifestyle.

   • *How will the frying or extra sugar, salt, peppers, and other flavorings to my food affect my quality of life (economically, physically, spiritually, socially, and mentally)—day to day?*

   • *How will reducing and/or avoiding the extra sugar, salt, peppers, and other flavorings to my food improve my quality of life (economically, physically, spiritually, socially, and mentally)—day to day?*

4.   Culture adds meaning to reality.

   • *How will the frying and extra food preparations that I add to my daily foods affect my weight?*

   • *How will changing how I prepare my foods affect my weight?*

5.   Culture is differently shared.

   • *How are the frying and my extra food preparations similar and/or different from other family members and friends?*

- *How are my reduced and/or avoidance of frying and extra food preparations similar and/or different from other family members and friends?*

6. Culture is adaptive.

- *How are my extra food preparations affecting who I am?*
- *How is my reduction and/or avoidance of frying and extra food preparations affecting who I am?*

Your answers to this set of six cultural health and fitness questions will most likely help you to not only recognize how you learned individual food preparation patterns (parents) but most importantly how your unhealthy food preparations (primarily adding sugar—"sweet tooth") were highly influenced by immediate social and familial environments. When faced with the reality that your preferred food preparations were causing you more and more health problems (cavities, skin, and face problems and too much extra energy), you will most likely take constructive steps in challenging and changing your food preparations from frying foods to baking foods (chicken and fish) and to using substitute food items such as sugar substitutes, sodium substitutes, and dairy substitutes (lactose added to milk products) that also benefit you nutritiously while still *tastin' good!*

Exercise

Because physical activity, fitness, and exercise play a vital role not only in losing weight but also in reducing your chances of developing chronic diseases such as hypertension, cancer, stroke, and diabetes, we must examine the physical activity patterns among African Americans and find out which fitness and exercise regimen truly works in all types of African American communities.

The *cultural health and physical fitness questions* that you may ask yourself are as follows:

1. Culture is learned.

- *How did I learn how to exercise?*
- *How am I going to start an exercise regimen that I prefer?*

2. Culture is transmitted by symbols.

- *How am I perceived by other family members and friends as a person who does not exercise or is not willing to try any physical activity?*
- *How am I perceived by other family members and friends as a person who exercises and maintains a physical fitness regimen?*

3. Culture is integrated in your total lifestyle.

    *   *How will the lack of exercise and any physical activity affect my quality of life (economically, physically, spiritually, socially, and mentally)—day to day?*

    *   *How will an exercise and physical fitness regimen improve my quality of life (economically, physically, spiritually, socially, and mentally)—day to day?*

4. Culture adds meaning to reality.

    *   *How will the lack of exercise and any physical activity affect my weight?*

    *   *How will developing or changing how I exercise the way I prefer affect my weight?*

5. Culture is differently shared.

    *   *How is my lack of exercise and lack of any physical activity similar and/or different from other family members and friends?*

    *   *How is my exercise and physical fitness regimen similar and/or different from other family members and friends?*

6. Culture is adaptive.

    *   *How is the lack of exercise and lack of any physical activity affecting who I am?*

    *   *How is my exercise and physical fitness regimen affecting who I am?*

Your answers to this set of six cultural health and physical fitness questions help you to not only recognize how you have learned your exercise regimen (sports and playing football) but, most importantly, how your exercise and physical fitness regimen must change as you get older. When faced with the reality that your preferred exercise and physical fitness regimen may cause more and more health problems (exhausation, increased muscle aches, increased muscle strains, and sprained ankles), you may have to take constructive steps in challenging and changing your exercise and physical fitness regimen by incorporating more walking, jogging, yoga, Tae-Bo, and low-impact football drills (back-peddling) to meet your desired culturally appropriate exercise and physical fitness regimen.

Summary

The four key elements to health and fitness—*body image, food selection, food preparation,* and *exercise*—are the focus of this book and the foundation to my New Black Cultural Diet™. Like everyone who is battling their weight problem and attempting to find a diet plan that works for them, I have designed a diet plan that works very well for me and I believe all of those who share my ethnic, social, historical, and cultural background. I felt that these four key elements to health and fitness provide the basis on which to challenge and to change the cultural preferences among African Americans regarding foods, dieting, and fitness.

By answering the cultural health and physical fitness questions, I discovered how my cultural issues (surface structure and deep structure) influenced my success or failure to sustain a health and fitness regimen. I also discovered that if I approached the health and fitness issue in a *culturally appropriate* way, then I could really uncover the *real reasons* why I had recurring problems with my weight. Over the years, the *real reasons* why I had problems with my weight were:

- Maintaining certain family and ethnic patterns of food selection (high consumption of pork and red meat products) and food preparation (foods high in sodium or adding table salt, sugar, and fried foods);
- Changing lifestyle pattern (new job, new city, new baby) caused disruption of my regular health, fitness, exercise, and food habits; and
- Being less informed on what is bad for my health.
- *I simply did not know!*

Fortunately, I stuck with my culture—*African American culture*—and discovered new ways to use all the various facets of it in providing me a new way to fight the ongoing overweight and fitness issue. The strategies that I used to address the four key elements to health and fitness were as follows:

Body Image
- Looked at pictures of myself when I was a competitive athlete (high school and college football years).
- Decided that I wanted my body to look similar to my competitive body as opposed to the larger, bloated overweight body.

Food Selection
- Became more selective in the type of foods that are healthier, fresher, and still within my particular soul food pattern.

- Socialized and ate with family members and friends who shared my similar food selection choices.
- Carried and consumed bottled water on a daily basis.

Food Preparation

- Baked all foods that were traditionally fried.
- Removed all extra fats and skins from meat products.
- Used sodium substitutes, sugar substitutes, fat-free non-stick cooking sprays, and lactose-free products.

Exercise

- Maintained weekly exercise regimens (days always the same).
- Stretched more often, walked, jogged, and/or participated in active sporting activity with family on a regular weekly basis.
- Used Tae-Bo tapes (Basic Training, Flex and Ultimate Boot Camp) and practiced my low-impact football drills—back peddling.

By doing it the *culturally appropriate* way, I am

- losing the weight that I want;
- having the body that I want;
- eating the foods that I want;
- preparing the foods the way I want; and
- exercising the way that I want.

Thus, instead of *customizing* my health, diet, and fitness regimen, I *culturalized* it to fit me—a 47-year-old African American man.

Conclusion

Well, there you have it—my cultural diet approach for African Americans. As you can tell, it is not a complicated approach and it does not involve a lot of new jargon or language that most people do not understand. It does not cost you any major amount—monetarily. It is straightforward and goes to the cultural core of why "we," African Americans, are having a difficult time with overweight and obesity. The medical and health consequences cannot be overlooked anymore because we are simply losing too many family members and friends to this very preventable health issue!

One of the major reasons why I wrote this book is to provide myself and others a strategy that happens to be *culturally based* and *culturally designed* to fit our particular African American perspectives on health, fitness, dieting, food, and exercise. I believe this African American perspective is desperately needed today because what we are talking about now is our survival, and we have no more time to waste.

Therefore, instead of blaming our culture, which a lot of people do when things do not go right in the African American community, I have used various aspects of our culture in helping us to address and solve many of the issues surrounding overweight and obesity in our diverse communities. That's why this book examined body image, body type, and body build from the African American perspective. That's why this book examined food practices and the cultural meaning of *soul food* from the African American perspective. That's why this book examined physical fitness and exercise from the African American perspective. Finally, that's why this book placed dieting, health, and physical fitness in an African American cultural framework.

By taking this *cultural approach* and *cultural perspective*, we can collectively work together in not only understanding comprehensively this critical health issue but also in developing new *culturally appropriate health and fitness programs* that work for all of us—not just a select few. If you feel the way that I do, then encourage others such as health and fitness experts, nutritionists, public health administrators, community-based organizers, physicians, nurses, health professionals, church leaders, union organization leaders, presidents of historically black colleges, fraternity and sorority leaders, politicians, researchers, extended family members, mothers, fathers, children, and even other anthropologists to do their part in solving this serious health epidemic.

So as I said at the beginning of this book, go ahead and design all the fancy and trendy diet and physical fitness programs that you can imagine. One thing is for sure, from my perspective, *culture* is the key in winning this battle of overweight and obesity not only in the African American community but also in all our communities!

Postevaluation Questions

1. Can most health professionals easily incorporate a cultural approach to a diet regimen?

   Most health professionals can easily incorporate a cultural approach to a diet regimen simply by taking the time to listen, to observe, to respect, and to conduct a little background research on the health patterns associated with their particular African American population.

2.   How can health professionals recognize the importance of cultural factors to African Americans' dietary pattern?

Health professionals will recognize the importance of cultural factors to African Americans' dietary pattern when they can see how many more African Americans will follow a healthier dietary regimen that includes more African American foods than those that do not.

3.   How can African Americans learn new approaches to losing weight and keeping it off?

African Americans can learn new approaches to losing weight and keeping it off by recognizing that they are not alone but always a part of a close network of family members and friends in their effort in losing weight and keeping it off.

References

American Institute for Cancer Research. 1997. *Food, Nutrition and Prevention of Cancer: A Global Perspective.* Washington, D.C.: World Cancer Research Fund.

Bailey, E. 1994. Medical anthropologist as health department consultant. *Practicing Anthropology* 16:13–15.

———. 2000. *Medical Anthropology and African American Health.* Westport, CT: Bergin & Garvey.

Brangman, S. 1995. African American elders: Implications for health care providers. *Clinics in Geriatric Medicine* 11:15–23.

Guidry, J., Mathews-Juarez, P., Copeland, V. 2003. Barriers to breast cancer control for African American women: The interdependence of culture and psychosocial issues. *Cancer* 97 (1 Suppl):318–323.

Jacobson, T., Morton, F., Jacobson, K., Sharma, S., and Garcia, D. 2002. An assessment of obesity among African American women in an inner city primary care clinic. *Journal of the National Medical Association* 94:1049–1057.

Jennings, K. 1996. Getting black women to screen for cancer: Incorporating health beliefs into practice. *Journal of the American Academy of Nursing Practitoners* 8:53–59.

Kittler, P., and Sucher, K. 2001. *Food and Culture.* Belmont, CA: Wadsworth Thomson Learning.

Martin, J., and Panicucci, C. 1996. Health-related practices and priorities: The health behaviors and beliefs of community-living black older women. *Journal of Gerontological Nursing* 22:41–48.

Mouton, C., Johnson, M., and Cole, D. 1995. Ethical considerations with African American elders. *Ethnogeriatics* 11:113–129.

Mouton, C., Harris, S., Rovi, S., Solorzano, P., and Johnson, M. 1997. Barriers to black women's participation in cancer clinical trials. *Journal of the National Medical Association* 89:721–727.

Pinn, V. 1996. Status of women's health research: Where are African American women? *Journal of National Black Nurses Association* Spring-Summer 8:8–19.

Price J. 1993. "Prostate cancer: Perceptions of African American males." *Journal of the National Medical Association* 85:941–947.

Robinson, T., and Killen, J. 2001. Obesity prevention for children and adolescents. In K. Thompson and L. Smolak (Eds.), *Body Image, Eating Disorders and Obesity in Youth*. Washington, DC: American Psychological Association, 261–292.

Rosenberg, L., Adams-Campbell, L., and Palmer, J. 1995. The black women's health study: A follow-up study for causes and preventions of illness. *Journal of American Medical Women's Association* 50:56–58.

Thompson, K., and Smolak, L. (Eds.). 2001. *Body Image, Eating Disorders and Obesity in Youth*. Washington, DC: American Psychological Association.

Stolley, M., and Fitzgibbon, M. 1997. Effects of an obesity prevention program on the eating behavior of African American mothers and daughters. *Health Education and Behavior* 24:152–164.

Walcott-McQuigg, J., Chen, S., Davis, K., Stevenson, E., Choi, A., Wangsrikhun, S. 2002. Weight loss and weight loss maintenance in African-American women. *Journal of the National Medical Association* 94:686–694.

Weinrich, S., Holdford, D., Boyd, M., Creanga, D., Johnson, A., Frank-Stromborg, M., and Weinrich, M. 1998. Prostate cancer education in African American churches. *Public Health Nursing* 15:188–195.

Whitehead, T. 1992. In search of soul food and meaning: Culture, food, and health. In H. Baer and Y. Jones (Eds.), *African Americans in the South: Issues of Race, Class and Gender*. Athens: The University of Georgia Press, 94–110.

Willet, W. 2001. *Eat, Drink, and Be Healthy: The Harvard Medical School Guide to Healthy Eating*. New York: Simon and Schuster.

U.S. Department of Health and Human Services. 1997. Health United States 1996–97. Washington, DC: National Center for Health Statistics. DHHS Publication No. 97-1232.

Appendix: Useful Sources

University Web sites

The University of California at Berkeley—Center for Weight and Health

http://nature.berkeley.edu/cwh/index.html
The mission of the Center for Weight and Health is to provide leadership for the development of science-based solutions to weight-related health problems, with a focus on children and their families.

East Carolina University—Growing Up FIT!

http://www.ncagromedicine.org/fit.htm
The Growing Up FIT! Program is an ongoing collaborative community partnership committed to developing sustainable programming to assist children to achieve and maintain a healthy weight. FIT! had developed innovative, culturally competent physical activity and food and nutrition education programming for Pitt County (North Carolina) Elementary School system.

Government Web sites

The National Cancer Institute at the National Institutes of Health—5 a Day Program for African Americans, African American Men, African American Women, and African American churches

http://5aday.gov/aahealth/index.html
http://5aday.gov/aahealth/aamen/index.html
http://5aday.gov/aahealth/aawomen/index.html

http://5aday.gov/aahealth/bodyandsoul/index.html
The 5 to 9 a Day for Better Health program encourages African Americans to eat more fruits and vegetables every day for better health and empowers African Americans to take charge of their health and gain access to vital health information.

The National Heart, Lung, and Blood Institute at the National Institutes of Health—Heart Healthy Home Cooking: African American Style booklet

http://www.nhlbi.nih.gov/health/public/heart/other/chdblack/cooking.htm
Prepare your favorite African American dishes in ways that protect you and your family from heart disease and stroke. These 20 tested recipes will show you how to cut back on saturated fat, cholesterol, salt, and sodium and still have great-tasting food. Delicious foods from spicy Southern barbecued chicken to sweet potato pie are included.

African American Health-Oriented Web sites

Black Women's Health

http://www.blackwomenshealth.com
This is an exciting, informative, and interactive Web site dedicated to promoting the physical, mental, and spiritual wellness of today's African American woman.

Fitness for the Urban Culture

http://www.pihpoh.com
This is a health-and-fitness Web site for the urban culture. They have made it their business to deliver the truth and nothing but the truth when it comes to health and fitness.

California Adolescent Nutrition and Fitness Program

http://www.canfit.org
The California Adolescent Nutrition and Fitness (CANFit) Program is a statewide, nonprofit organization whose mission is to engage communities and build their capacity to improve the nutrition and physical activity status of California's low-income African American, American Indian, Latino, Asian American, and Pacific Islander youth 10–14 years old.

African American Diet and Physical Fitness Books

Slim Down Sister: The African American Woman's Guide to Healthy, Permanent Weight Loss by Roniece Weaver, Fabiola Gaines, and Angela Ebron. 2001. Plume Books.

Slim Down Sister offers a comprehensive program of diet and exercise especially geared to empower African American women to take control of their weight and their health. This unique book, written by experts in the fields of health and nutrition, shares important information about losing weight and keeping it off; reducing the risk of diabetes, hypertension, and heart disease; and many more helpful dietary tips.

Dr. Ro's Ten Secrets to Livin' Healthy by Rovenia Brock. 2003. Bantam.

From the "Big Ten" myths about miracle weight loss diets to how eating the right foods can help you live longer and why soul food (if prepared properly) really can be good for you, Dr. Ro shows how serious illnesses can be largely prevented.

Work It Out: The Black Woman's Guide to Getting the Body You Always Wanted by MaDonna Grimes. 2003. Avery Publishing Group.

In *Work It Out*, fitness expert MaDonna Grimes offers black women a different ideal to work toward suited to their unique physiques. Drawing from her experience as a professional dancer, choreographer, and fitness competitor, Grimes has fashioned a revolutionary program specifically for black women to help them attain their fitness goals and build self-esteem. Her dynamic, innovative plan includes African and Afro-Latin dance moves, weight training, stretching, and proper nutrition. She also addresses health issues common to black women, such as obesity, hypertension, and diabetes, and explains how they can be avoided with proper nutrition and exercise.

Physical Fitness Programs

Tae Bo®

http://www.billyblanks.com

Tae Bo is a program that combines the best of a variety of different exercise disciplines in an overall workout. It is a combination of the self-awareness and control of martial arts, the force of boxing, and the grace and rhythm of dance.

24 Hour Fitness®

http://www.24hourfitness.com

24 Hour Fitness, the world's largest privately owned and operated fitness center chain, began as a one-club operation in 1983. The vision of 24 Hour Fitness is to make fitness a way of life by creating the ultimate in multisport fitness centers and make them affordable and accessible to people of all abilities and fitness levels.

Bally Total Fitness

http://opal.ballyfitness.com

The mission of Bally Total Fitness is to be a total fitness resource by providing quality service and outstanding fitness your way. Bally Total Fitness combines dynamic personal training, basic nutrition education, and a new personalized online weight-loss program.

Gold's Gym

http://www.goldsgym.com

Gold's Gym has been in fitness since 1965, dating back to the original Gold's Gym in Venice, California. Today, Gold's Gym has expanded its fitness profile to offer all of the latest equipment and services including group exercise, personal training, cardiovascular equipment, spinning, Pilates, and yoga, while maintaining its core weight-lifting tradition.

BIBLIOGRAPHY

Airhihenbuwa, C. O., S. Kumanyika, T. Agurs, and A. Lowe. "Perceptions and Beliefs about Exercise, Rest, and Health among African Americans." *American Journal of Health Promotion* 9 (1995): 426–429.

Airhihenbuwa, C. O., S. Kumanyika, T. Agurs, A. Lowe, D. Saunders, and C. Morssink. "Cultural Aspects of African American Eating Patterns." *Ethnicity and Health* 1 (1996): 245–260.

Allison, D., K. Fontaine, J. Manson, J. Stevens, and T. VanItallie. "Annual Deaths Attributable to Obesity in the United States." *Journal of the American Medical Association* 282 (1999): 1530–1538.

Altabe, M. "Ethnicity and Body Image: Quantitative and Qualitative Analysis." *International Journal of Eating Disorders* 23 (1998): 153–159.

American Cancer Society. Cancer Facts and Figures–1998. Atlanta, GA: American Cancer Society, 1998.

American Diabetes Association. Press Conference, August 8, 2001.

American Institute for Cancer Research. *Food, Nutrition and Prevention of Cancer: A Global Perspective.* Washington, DC: World Cancer Research Fund, 1997.

Aschenbrenner, J. "Extended Families among Black Americans." *Journal of Comparative Family Studies* 4 (1973): 257–268.

Babey, S., A. Diamant, R. Brown, and T. Hastert. "California Adolescents Increasing Inactive." *UCLA Health Policy Research Brief* April (2005): 1–7.

Bailey, E. "Black Female Parents and Stress." *Psychological Reports* 55 (1984): 927–931.

———. "Medical Anthropologist as Health Department Consultant." *Practicing Anthropology* 16 (1994): 13–15.

———. *Medical Anthropology and African American Health.* Westport, CT: Bergin & Garvey, 2000.

Base-Smith, V., and J. Campinha-Bacote. "The Culture of Obesity." *Journal of National Black Nurses Association* 14, no. 1 (2003): 52–56.

Baskin, M., H. Ahluwalia, and K. Resnicow. "Obesity Intervention among African American Children and Adolescents." *Pediatric Clinics of North America* 48 (2001): 1027–1039.

Becker, D., L. Yanek, D. Koffman, and Y. Bronner. "Body Image Preferences among Urban African Americans and Whites from Low Income Communities. *Ethnicity and Disease* 9 (1999): 377–386.

Belza, B., J. Walwick, S. Shiu-Thornto, S. Schwartz, M. Taylor, and J. Lo Gerfo. "Older Adult Perspectives on Physical Activity and Exercise: Voices From Multiple Cultures." *Preventing Chronic Disease 1*, no. 4 (2004): 1–11.

Brangman, S. "African American Elders: Implications for Health Care Providers." *Clinics in Geriatric Medicine* 11 (1995): 15–23.

Brown, P., and M. Konner. "An Anthropological Perspective on Obesity." *Annals of the New York Academy of Sciences* 499 (1987): 29–46.

Burton, B., W. Foster, J. Hirsch, and T. Van Itallie. "Health Implications of Obesity: NIH Consensus Development Conference." *International Journal of Obesity and Related Metabolic Disorders* 9 (1985): 155–169.

Cachelin, F., R. Rebeck, G. Chung., and E. Pelayo. "Does Ethnicity Influence Body-Size Preference? A Comparison of Body Image and Body Size." *Obesity Research* 10 (2002): 158–166.

Campbell, M., W. Dmark-Wahnefried, M. Symons, W. Kalsbeek, J. Doods, A. Cowan, B. Jackson, B. Motsinger, K. Hoben, J. Lashley, S. Demissie, and J. McClelland. "Fruit and Vegetable Consumption and Prevention of Cancer: The Black Churches United for Better Health Project." *American Journal of Public Health* 89 (1999): 1390–1396.

Caspersen, C., and R. Merritt. "Trends in Physical Activity Patterns among Older Adults: The Behavioral Risk Factor Surveillance System, 1986–1990." *Medicine and Science in Sports and Exercise* 24, suppl. (1992): S26.

CBS2-New York. Bill Clinton Joins Child Obesity Fight, 2005. http:cbsnewyork .com/healthwatch/health_story_123150452.html.

Centers for Disease Control and Prevention. DATA2010. Healthy People 2010 Database, 2004. http://www.wonder.cdc.gov/DATA2010.

Centers for Disease Control and Prevention. Physical Activity for Everyone: Physical Activity Terms, 2005. http://www.cdc.gov/nccdphp/ dnpa/physical/terms/index.htm.
Physical Activity and Public Health. http://wonder.cdc.gov/wonder/ prevguid/p0000391/p0000391.asp.

Centers for Disease Control and Prevention. The National Center for Health Statistics. "Obesity Still on the Rise, New Data Show," 2002. http:// www.cdc.gov/nchs/releases/02news/obesityonrise.htm.

Centers for Disease Control and Prevention. The National Center for Chronic Disease Prevention and Health Promotion. "Basics about Overweight and Obesity," 2002. http://www.cdc.gov/nccdphp/ dnpa/obesity/basics.htm.

Clinton Foundation Organization. Press Release: Clinton Foundation and American Heart Association Form Alliance to Create a Healthier Generation, 2005.

http:www.clintonfoundation.org/050305-nr-cf-hs-pr-wjc-and-american-heart-association-healthier-generation-initiative.htm.

Daniels, S., D. Arnett, R. Eckel, S. Gidding, L. Hayman, S. Kumanyika, T. Robinson, B. Scott, S. Jeor, and C. Williams. "Overweight in Children and Adolescents: Pathophysiology, Consequences, Prevention, and Treatment." *Circulation* 111 (2005): 1999–2012.

Davis, E., J. Clark, J. Carrese, T. Gary, and L. Cooper. "Racial and Socioeconomic Differences in the Weight-Loss Experiences of Obese Women." *American Journal of Public Health* 95, no. 9 (2005): 1539–1543.

Delany, S., E. A. Delany, and A. H. Hearth. *The Delany Sisters' Book of Everyday Wisdom*. New York: Kodansh International, 1994.

Desmond, S., J. Price, R. Lock, D. Smith, and P. Stewart. "Urban Black and White Adolescents' Physical Fitness Status and Perceptions of Exercise." *Journal of School Health* 60 (1990): 220–226.

DiPietro, L., and C. Caspersen. "National Estimates of Physical Activity among White and Black Americans." *Medicine and Science in Sports and Exercise* 23, suppl. (1991): S105.

Dirks, R., and N. Duran. "African American Dietary Patterns at the Beginning of the 20th Century." *Journal of Nutrition* 131 (2001): 1881–1889.

Dixon, B., and J. Wilson. *Good Health for African Americans*. New York: Crown Publishers, 1994.

Dounchis, J., H. Hayden, and D. Wilfley. "Obesity, Body Image and Eating Disorders in Ethnically Diverse Children and Adolescents." In *Body Image, Eating Disorders and Obesity in Youth*, edited by K. Thompson and L. Smolak Washington, DC: American Psychological Association, 2001.

Esposito, K., A. Pontillo, C. Di Palo, G. Giugliano, M. Masella, R. Marfella, and D. Giugliano. "Effect of Weight Loss and Lifestyle Changes on Vascular Inflammatory Markers in Obese Women: A Randomized Trial." *Journal of the American Medical Association* 289 (2003): 1799–1804.

Etkin, S., D. Lenker, and Mills, E. J. *Professional Guide to Diseases*. Springhouse, PA: Springhouse, 1998.

Farmer, M., T. Harris, J. Madans, R. Wallace, J. Cornoni-Huntley, and L. White. "The NHANES I Epidemiologic Follow-up Study." *Journal of the American Geriatric Society* 37, no. 1 (1989): 9–16.

Fieldhouse, P. *Food and Nutrition: Customs and Culture*. Second ed. New York: Chapman & Hall, 1992.

Flegal, K., M. Carrol, C. Ogden, and C. Johnson. "Prevalence and Trends in Obesity among U.S. Adults, 1999–2000." *Journal of the American Medical Association* 288 (2002): 1723–1727.

Flores, G., E. Fuentes-Afflick, O. Barbot, O. Carter-Pokras, L. Claudio, M. Lara, J. McLaurin, L. Pachter, F. Gomez, F. Mendoza, R.Valdez, A. Villarruel, R. Zambrana, R. Greenberg, and M. Weitzman. "The Health of Latino Children: Urgent Priorities, Unanswered Questions, and a Research Agenda." *Journal of the American Medical Association* 288 (2002): 82–90.

Fontanarosa, P. "Obesity Research: A Call for Papers." *Journal of the American Medical Association* 288 (2002): 1772–1773.

Fox, K. "The Influence of Physical Activity on Mental Well-Being in the Community." *Public Health Nutrition* 2-3A (1999): 411–418.

Franklin, J., and A. Moss. *From Slavery to Freedom: A History of Negro Americans.* New York: Alfred A. Knopf, 1988.

Garnett, C. "Panel Weighs In on Diet, Fat & Cholesterol." *The NIH Record.* 54 (2002): 1, 8–9.

Gary, T., K. Baptiste-Roberts, E. Gregg, D. Williams, G. Beckles, E. Miller, and M. Engelgau. "Fruit, Vegetable and Fat Intake in a Population-Based Sample of African Americans." *Journal of the National Medical Association* 96, no. 12 (2004): 1599–1605.

Gillum, R. "Overweight and Obesity in Black Women: A Review of Published Data from the National Center for Health Statistics." *Journal of the National Medical Association* 79 (1987): 865–871.

Giovannucci, E., A. Ascherio, E. Rimm, G. Colditz, M. Stampfer, and W. Willett. "Physical Activity, Obesity, and Risk for Colon Cancer and Adenoma in Men." *Annals of Internal Medicine* 122, no. 5 (1995): 327–334.

Gordon-Larsen, P., L. Adair, and B. Popkin. "The Relationship of Ethnicity, Socioeconomic Factors, and Over-weight in U.S. Adolescents." *Obesity Research* 11, no. 1 (2003): 121–129.

Gore, S. "African American Women's Perceptions of Weight: Paradigm Shift for Advanced Practice." *Holistic Nursing Practice* 13 (1999): 71–79.

Gordon-Larsen, P., P. Griffiths, M. Bentley, D. Ward, K. Kelsey, K. Shields, and A. Ammerman. "Barriers to Physical Activity: Qualitative Data on Caregiver-Daughter Perceptions and Practices." *American Journal of Preventive Medicine* 27, no. 3 (2004): 218–223.

Grimes, M. *Work It Out: The Black Women's Guide to Getting the Body You Always Wanted.* New York: Penguin Putnam, 2003.

Guidry, J. et al. "Cultural Sensitivity and Readability of Breast and Prostate Printed Cancer Education Materials Targeting African Americans." *Journal of the National Medical Association* 90 (1998): 165–169.

Hu, F., M. Stampfer, G. Colditz, A. Ascherio, K. Rexrode, W. Willett, and J. Manson. "Physical Activity and Risk of Stroke in Women." *Journal of the American Medical Association* 283, no. 22 (2000): 2961–2967.

Hu, F., J. Manson, M. Stampfer, G. Colditz, S. Liu, C. Solomon, and W. Willett. "Diet, Lifestyle, and the Risk of Type 2 Diabetes Mellitus in Women." *New England Journal of Medicine* 345, no. 11 (2001): 790–797.

Jacobson, T., F. Morton, K. Jacobson, S. Sharma, and D. Garcia. "An Assessment of Obesity among African American Women in an Inner City Primary Care Clinic." *Journal of the National Medical Association* 94 (2002): 1049–1057.

Jennings, K. "Getting Black Women to Screen for Cancer: Incorporating Health Beliefs Into Practice." *Journal of the American Academy of Nursing Practitoners* 8 (1996): 53–59.

Joshipura, K., A. Ascherio, J. Manson, M. Stampfer, E. Rimm, F. Speizer, C. Hennekens, D. Spiegelman, and W. Willet. "Fruit and Vegetable Intake in Relation to Risk of Ischemic Stroke." *Journal of the American Medical Association* 282 (1999): 1233–1239.

Kanders, B., P. Ullman-Joy, J. Foreyt, S. Heymsfield, D. Heber, R. Elashoff, J. Ashley, R. Reeves, and G. Blackburn. "The Black American Lifestyle Intervention (BALI): The Design of a Weight Loss Program for Working-Class African American Women." *Journal of the American Dietetic Association* 94 (1994): 310–312.

Kittler, P., and K. Sucher. *Food and Culture.* Belmont, CA: Wadsworth Thomson Learning, 2001.

Kris-Etherton, P., R. Eckle, B. Howard, S. St. Jeor, and T. Bazzarre. "Lyon Diet Program/American Heart Association Step I Dietary Pattern on Cardiovascular Disease." *Circulation* 103 (2001): 1823–1825.

Kumanyika, S., C. Morssink, and T. Agurs. "Models for Dietary and Weight Change in African American Women: Identifying Cultural Components." *Ethnicity and Disease* 2 (1992): 166–175.

LaBelle, P. *LaBelle Cuisine: Recipes to Sing About.* New York: Broadway Books, 1999.

Lavizzo-Mourey, R., C. Cox, N. Strumpf, W. Edwards, R. Lavizzo-Mourey, M. Stineman, and J. A. Grisso. "Attitudes and Beliefs about Exercise among Elderly African Americans in an Urban Community." *Journal of the National Medical Association* 93 (2001): 475–480.

Martin, J., and C. Panicucci. "Health-Related Practices and Priorities: The Health Behaviors and Beliefs of Community-Living Black Older Women." *Journal of Gerontological Nursing* 22 (1996): 41–48.

McKeever, C., C. Faddis, N. Koroloff, and J. Henn. "Wellness Within REACH: Mind, Body, and Soul: A No-Cost Physical Activity Program for African Americans in Portland, Oregon to Combat Cardiovascular Disease." *Ethnicity and Disease* 14 (Summer 2004): S1-93–S1-101.

McTigue, K., J. Garrett, and B. Popkin. "The Natural History of the Development of Obesity in a Cohort of Young U.S. Adults between 1981 and 1998." *Annals of Internal Medicine* 136 (2002): 857–864.

Meyers, R., T. Wolf, A. Balshem, E. Ross, and G. Chodak. "Receptivity of African American Men to Prostate Cancer Screening." *Urology* 43 (1994): 480–487.

Michigan Department of Community Health. An Epidemic of Overweight and Obesity in Michigan's African American Women, 2002. www .michigan.gov/documents/Healthy_Michigan_2010_1_88117_7.pdf.

Miller, K., D. Gleaves, T. Hirsch, B. Green, A. Snow, and C. Corbett. "Comparisons of Body Image Dimensions by Race/Ethnicity and Gender in a University Population." *International Journal of Eating Disorders* 27 (2000): 310–316.

Mitchell, T. "Keep Moving Toward the Lite." *USA Weekend.* November 15–17 (2002): 6–11.

Mokdad, A., M. Serdula, W. Dietz, B. Bowman, J. Marks, and J. Koplan. "The Spread of the Obesity Epidemic in the United States, 1991–1998." *Journal of the American Medical Association* 282 (1999): 1519–1522.

Mouton, C., M. Johnson, and D. Cole. "Ethical Considerations with African American Elders." *Ethnogeriatics* 11 (1995): 113–129.

Mouton, C., S. Harris, S. Rovi, P. Solorzano, and M. Johnson. "Barriers to Black Women's Participation in Cancer Clinical Trials." *Journal of the National Medical Association* 89 (1997): 721–727.

Must, A., J. Spadano, E. Coakley, A. Field, G. Colditz, and W. Dietz. "The Disease Burden Associated with Overweight and Obesity." *Journal of the American Medical Association* 282 (1999): 1523–1529.

National Cancer Institute. *Fruits and Vegetables: Men Eat 9 a Day.* Washington, DC: NIH Publication:03-5332, 2003. http://5aday.gov/ 9aday/blackmen-shealth/diet/diet.html.

National Center for Health Statistics. *Health United States 1996–97 and Injury Chartbook.* Hyattsville, MD (1997): DHHS Publication PHS 97-1232.

National Council of Negro Women. *The Black Family Reunion Cookbook.* New York: Fireside Books, 1991.

National Heart, Lung, and Blood Institute. National Institutes of Health. *Clinical Guidelines on the Identification, Evaluation, and Treatment of Overweight and Obesity in Adults: Executive Summary.* Hyattsville, MD (1998): DHHS Publication PHS 98-4083.

National Institute of Diabetes and Digestive Disorders.. *Sisters Together: Move More, Eat Better Program,* 2003. http://www.niddk.nih.gov.

National Institutes of Health. *Heart Healthy Home Cooking: African American Style.* Washington, DC (1997): NIH Publication 97-3792.

Neumar-Sztainer, D., M. Story, P. Hannan, and J. Croll. "Overweight Status and Eating Patterns Among Adolescents: Where Do Youths Stand in Comparison with the Healthy People 2010 Objectives." *American Journal of Public Health* 92 (2002): 844–851.

Nichols, D., C. Sanborn, S. Bonnick, V. Ben Ezra, B. Gench, and N. DiMarco. "The Effects of Gymnastics Training on Bone Mineral Density." *Medicine and Science in Sports and Exercise* 26, no. 10 (1994): 1220–1225.

Nies, M., M. Vollman, and T. Cook. "African American Women's Experience with Physical Activity in their Daily Lives." *Public Health Nursing* 16 (1999): 23–31.

Ogden, C., K. Flegal, M. Carroll, and C. Johnson. "Prevalence and Trends in Overweight Among U.S. Children and Adolescents, 1999–2000." *Journal of the American Medical Association* 288 (2002): 1728–1732.

Olshansky, S., D. Passaro, R. Hershow, J. Layden, B. Carnes, J. Brody, L. Hayflick, R. Butler, D. Allison, and D. Ludwig. "A Potential Decline in Life Expectancy in the United States in the 21st Century." *New England Journal of Medicine* 352, no. 11 (2005): 1138–1145.

Paffenbarger, R., R. Hyde, A. Wing, and C. Steinmetz. "A Natural History of Athleticism and Cardiovascular Health." *Journal of the American Medical Association* 252, no. 4 (1984): 491–495.

Parker, S., M. Nichter, M. Nichter, S. C. Vuckovic, and C. Ritenbaugh. "Body Image and Weight Concerns among African American and White Adolescent Females: Differences that Make a Difference." *Human Organization* 54 (1995): 103–114.

Paschal, A, R. Lewis, A. Martin, D. Dennis-Shipp, and D. Simpson. "Baseline Assessment of the Health Status and Health Behaviors of African Americans

Participating in the Activities for Life Program: A Community-Based Health Intervention Program." *Journal of Community Health* 29, no. 4 (2004): 305–318.

Pate, R. M. Pratt, S. Blair, W. Haskell, C. Macera, C. Bouchard, D. Buchner, W. Ettinger, G. Heath, and A. King. "Physical Activity and Public Health. A Recommendation from the Centers for Disease Control and Prevention and the American College of Sports Medicine." *Journal of the American Medical Association* 273, no. 5 (1995): 402–407.

Patterson, B., L. Harlan, G. Block, and L. Kahle. "Food Choices of Whites, Blacks, and Hispanics: Data from the 1987 National Health Interview Survey." *Nutrition and Cancer* 23 (1995): 105–119.

Pinn, V. "Status of Women's Health Research: Where Are African American Women?" *Journal of National Black Nurses Association* 8, no. 1 (1995): 8–19.

Price, J., T. Colvin, and D. Smith. "Prostate Cancer: Perceptions of African American Males." *Journal of the National Medical Association* 85 (1993): 941–947.

Pulvers, K., R. Lee, H. Kaur, M. Mayo, M. Flitzgibbon, S. Jeffries, J. Butler, Q. Hou, and J. Ahluwalia. "Development of a Culturally Relevant Body Image Instrument among Urban African Americans." *Obesity Research* 12, no. 10 (2004): 1641–1651.

Ransdell, L., and C. Wells. "Physical Activity in Urban White, African American, and Mexican American Women." *Medicine and Science in Sports and Exercise* 30 (1998): 1608–1615.

Robertson, R., and L. Smaha. "Can a Mediterranean-Style Diet Reduce Heart Disease?" *Circulation* 103 (2001): 1821–1822.

Robinson, T., and J. Killen. "Obesity Prevention for Children and Adolescents." In *Body Image, Eating Disorders and Obesity in Youth*, edited by K. Thompson and L. Smolak. Washington, DC: American Psychological Association, 2001.

Robinson, T., J. Chang, K. Haydel, and J. Killen. "Overweight Concerns and Body Dissatisfaction among Third-Grade Children: The Impacts of Ethnicity and Socioeconomic Status." *Journal of Pediatrics* 138 (2001): 181–187.

Rosenberg, L., L. Adams-Campbell, and J. Palmer. "The Black Women's Health Study: A Follow-Up Study for Causes and Preventions of Illness." *Journal of American Medical Women's Association* 50 (1995): 56–58.

Satcher, D. "Overweight and Obesity Threatens U.S. Health Gains." U.S. Department of Health and Human Services Press Release, Thursday, December 31, 2001. http://www.surgeongeneral.gov/news/pressreleases/pr_obesity.htm.

Satia, J., J. Glanko, and A. Siega-Riz. "Eating at Fast-Food Restaurants is Associated with Dietary Intake, Demographic, Psychosocial and Behavioural Factors among African Americans in North Carolina." *Public Health Nutrition* 7, no. 8 (2004): 1089–1096.

Schlundt, D., M. Hargreaves, and M. Buchowski. "The Eating Behavior Patterns Questionnaire Predicts Dietary Fat Intake in African American Women." *Journal of the American Dietetic Association* 103 (2003): 338–345.

Schoenborn, C. A. "Health Habits of U.S. Adults, 1985: The Alameda 7 Revisited." *Public Health Reports* 101 (1986): 571–580.

Shavers, V., and S. Shankar. "Trend in the Prevalence of Overweight and Obesity among Urban African American Hospital Employees and Public Housing Residents." *Journal of the National Medical Association* 94 (2002): 566–576.

Simopoulos, A. "The Relationship Between Diet and Hypertension." *Complementary Therapy* 16 (1990): 25–30.

Singh, R., G. Dubnov, M. Niaz, S. Ghosh, R. Sing, S. Rastogi, O. Manor, D. Pella, and E. Berry. "Effect of an Indo-Mediterranean Diet on Progression of Coronary Artery Disease in High Risk Patients (Indo-Mediterranean Diet Heart Study): A Randomised Single-Blind Trial." *Lancet* 360 (2002): 1455–1461.

Smolak, L., and M. Levine. "Body Image in Children." In *Body Image, Eating Disorders and Obesity in Youth*, edited by K. Thompson and L. Smolak. Washington, DC: American Psychological Association, 2001.

Stack, C. *All Our Kin: Strategies for Survival in a Black Community*. New York: Harper & Row, 1974.

Staples, R. "Towards a Sociology of the Black Family: A Theoretical and Methodological Assessment." *Journal of Marriage and Family* 33 (1971): 19–138.

Stephens, T. "Secular Trends in Adult Physical Activity." *Research Quarterly in Exercise and Sports* 58 (1987): 94–105.

Stephens, T., D. Jacobs, and C. White. "A Descriptive Epidemiology of Leisure-Time Physical Activity." *Public Health Reports* 100 (1985): 147–158.

Stevens, J., S. Kumanyika, and J. Keil. "Attitudes toward Body Size and Dieting: Differences between Elderly Black and White Women." *American Journal of Public Health* 84 (1994): 1322–1325.

Stolley, M., and M. Fitzgibbon. "Effects of an Obesity Prevention Program on the Eating Behavior of African American Mothers and Daughters." *Health Education and Behavior* 24 (1997): 152–164.

Thompson, K., and L. Smolak, eds. *Body Image, Eating Disorders and Obesity in Youth*. Washington, DC: American Psychological Association, 2001.

Thompson, V., T. Baranowski, K. Cullen, L. Rittenberry, J. Baranowski, W. Taylor, and T. Nicklas. "Influences on Diet and Physical Activity among Middle-Class African American 8- to 10-Year-Old Girls at Risk of Becoming Obese." *Journal of Nutrition Education and Behavior* 35 (2003): 115–123.

Troiano, R., and K. Flegal. "Overweight Children and Adolescents: Description, Epidemiology, and Demographics." *Pediatrics* 101, no. 3 (1998): 497–504.

Troiano, R., K. Flegal, R. Kuczmarski, S. Campbell, and C. Johnson. "Overweight Prevalence and Trends for Children and Adolescents: The National Health and Nutrition Examination Surveys, 1963 to 1991." *Archives of Pediatric Adolescent Medicine* 149 (1995): 1085–1091.

U.S. Department of Health and Human Services. *Physical Activity and Health: A Report of the Surgeon General*. Atlanta, GA: U.S. Department of Health and

Human Services, Centers for Disease Control and Prevention, National Center for Chronic Disease and Prevention and Health Promotion, 1996.

——. *Health. United States 1996–97 and Injury Chartbook.* National Center for Health Statistics. Washington, DC: U.S. Government Printing Office, 1997. DHHS Publication 97-1232.

——. *Healthy People 2010*, 2nd ed. Washington, DC: U.S. Government Printing Office, 2000.

——. HHS Launches African American Obesity Initiative. U.S. DHHS. Office of Minority Health Press Release, 2005. http://www.os.dhhs.gov/news/press/2005pres/20050407.html.

USA Today. "Americans Urged to Exercise More, Eat Better," 2002. http://www.usatoday.com/news/health/2002-0-05-diet-guidelines_x.htm.

USA Today. "CDC Tries to Get Americans to Exercise," 2003 http://www.usatoday.com/news/health/2003-04-07-cdc-exercise_x.htm.

Veal, Y. "African Americans and Diabetes: Reasons, Rationale, and Research." *Journal of the National Medical Association* 88 (1996): 203–204.

Wagner, D., and V. Heyward. "Measures of Body Composition in Blacks and Whites: A Comparative Review." *American Journal of Clinical Nutrition* 71 (2000): 1392–1402.

Walcott-McQuigg, J., J. Sullivan, A. Dan, and B. Logan. "Psychosocial Factors Influencing Weight Control Behavior of African American Women." *Western Journal of Nursing Research* 17 (1995): 502–520.

Walcott-McQuigg, J., S. P. Chen, K. Davis, E. Stevenson, A. Choi, and W. Suparat. "Weight Loss and Weight Loss Maintenance in African American Women." *Journal of the National Medical Association* 94 (2002): 686–694.

Ward, D., S. Trost, G. Felton, R. Saunders, M. Parsons, M. Dowda, and R. Pate. "Physical Activity and Physical Fitness in African American Girls with and Without Obesity." *Obesity Research* 5 (1997): 572–577.

Weaver, R., F. Gaines, and A. Ebron. *Slim Down Sister: The African American Woman's Guide to Healthy, Permanent Weight Loss.* New York: Dutton, 2000.

Weinrich, S., D. Holdford, M. Boyd, D. Creanga, A. Johnson, M. Frank-Stromborg, and M. Weinrich. "Prostate Cancer Education in African American Churches." *Public Health Nursing* 15 (1998): 188–195.

Welch, C. S. Gross, Y. Bronner, D. Dewberry-Moore, and D. Paige. "Discrepancies in Body Image Perception among Fourth-Grade Public School Children from Urban, Suburban, and Rural Maryland." *Journal of the American Dietetic Association* 1040 (2004): 1080–1085.

White, C., K. Powell, G. Goelin, E. Gentry, and M. Forman. "The Behavioral Risk Factor Surveys, IV: The Descriptive Epidemiology of Exercise." *American Journal of Preventive Medicine* 3 (1987): 304–310.

Whitehead, T. "In Search of Soul Food and Meaning: Culture, Food, and Health." In *African Americans in the South: Issues of Race, Class and Gender,* edited by H. Baer and Y. Jones. Athens: University of Georgia Press, 1992.

Willet, W. *Eat, Drink, and Be Healthy: The Harvard Medical School Guide to Healthy Eating.* New York: Simon and Schuster, 2001.

Woods, J. *Soul Food: Recipes and Reflections from African American Churches.* New York: Harper Collins, 1998.

Woods, S., and Family. *Sylvia's Family Soul Food Cookbook: From Hemingway, South Carolina, to Harlem.* New York: William Morrow and Company, 1999.

Yancey, A., S. Kumanyika, N. Ponce, W. McCarthy, J. Fielding, J. Leslie, and J. Akbar. "Population-Based Interventions Engaging Communities of Color in Healthy Eating and Active Living: A Review." *Preventing Chronic Disease: Public Health Research, Practice, and Policy* 1, no. 1 (2004): 1–24.

Yanek, L., D. Becker, T. Moy, J. Gittelsohn, and D. Koffman. "Project Joy: Faith Based Cardiovascular Health Promotion for African American Women." *Public Health Reports*, 116, suppl. 1 (2001): 68–81.

Young. D., K. Miller, L. Wilder, L. Yanek, and D. Becker. "Physical Activity Patterns of Urban African Americans. *Journal of Community Health* 23 (1998): 99–112.

Young, D., J. Gittelsohn, J. Charleston, K. Felix-Aaron, and L. Appel. "Motivations for Exercise and Weight Loss Among African American Women: Focus Group Results and Their Contribution Towards Program Development." *Ethnicity and Health* 6 (2001): 227–245.

INDEX

African American adolescents, 52–54; exercise and physical fitness, 87–89

African American body image, 43–58; of adolescents, 52–54; of adults, 55–57; of children, 49–52; of college students, 54–55; of men, 55–57; of women, 55–57

African American cuisine, 66–70. *See also* Cultural history of African American cuisine

African American culture, 147

African American families, 4

African American family, 111–112

African American food habits, 64–66. *See also* Food habits, among African Americans

African American Health Belief Inventory (AAHBI), 16

Airhihenbuwa, Kumanyika, Agurs, Lowe, Saunders, and Morssink, 64–66

Anthropology, 107

Applied Medical Anthropology study, 7–13

Aschenbrenner, J., 111

Asian Americans, 49

Attributes of culture, 107, 140

Atwater, W. O., 68–69. *See also* USDA's Office of Experiment Stations

Bailey, Eric, 7, 107, 112

Behavioral Risk Factor Surveillance System (BRFSS), 26

Black America Lifestyle Intervention (BALI), 112–113

Body image, 43, 48, 141–142, 147; preferences among African Americans, 43–58. *See also* African American body image

Body mass index, 45, 46–48

Body type, 48–49

California Health Interview Survey, 87

CBS2 News, 28

Centers for Disease Control and Prevention, 25, 81–83

Childhood obesity, 28

Church culture, 114–116

Clinton, Bill, 28. *See also* William Clinton Foundation

Contemporary food habits, 70–72

Cultural approach, 34, 119, 149
Cultural appropriateness, 132, 138
Culturalized, 131, 148
Culturally appropriate, 113
Culturally appropriate health intervention strategies, 133–140. *See also* Culture and African American elderly; Culture and African American men; Culture and African American adolescent females; Culture and African American women
Culturally based, 20, 113
Culturally designed, 20
Cultural-dietary pattern, 106
Cultural health and physical fitness questions, 140–150
Cultural history of African American cuisine, 66–70
Culture, 107, 124, 149
Culture and African American elderly, 133. *See also* Culturally appropriate health intervention strategies
Culture and African American men, 135–136. *See also* Culturally appropriate health intervention strategies
Culture and African American adolescent females, 135–138. *See also* Culturally appropriate health intervention strategies
Culture and African American women, 134–135. *See also* Culturally appropriate health intervention strategies
Culture of obesity, 35

Davis, Esa, 16
Deep structural cultural components, 139–140
Delany Sisters, 83–84
Diabetes Mellitus, 5
Diabetes Study and African Americans, 7–13
Dietary patterns of African Americans, 62–64
Dirks and Duran, 68–70

Distinctive qualities of anthropology, 107
Dr. Tedd, 3

Eckel, Robert, 28
Ethnic minority groups, 26
European Americans, 12–13, 33, 48
Exercise, 82, 145–146, 148
Exercise and physical fitness among African Americans, 81–101

Federal programs, 110–123. *See also Fruits and Vegetables: Men Eat 9 a Day*; *Heart Healthy Home Cooking*; National Cancer Institute's 5 A Day Program; Sisters Together
Filipino, 49
Flexible cultural definition of healthiness, 44
Food, 64, 142
Food habits, 64, 142; among African Americans, 64–66. *See also* African American food habits
Food preferences among African Americans, 61–78
Food preparation, 144–145, 148
Food selection, 142–143, 147–148
Fruits and Vegetables: Men Eat 9 a Day, 122–123. *See also* Federal programs

Gerberding, Julie, 86
Good Health for African Americans, 123–124
Grimes, MaDonna, 85–86

Healthy Lifestyle Initiative, 14–16
Heart-Healthy Home Cooking, 119–120. *See also* Federal programs
Herman, Alexis, 78
Hispanics, 24, 26, 30, 48
Huckabee, Mike, 28

Indiana University Diabetes Research and Training Center, 7

"Keep Moving Toward the Lite," 3
Kittler and Sucher, 68–70
Kumanyika, Morrsink, and Agurs, 108–110

LaBelle, Patty, 76–77
Latinos, 24, 26, 30, 48
Leisure–time physical activity, 82
Lifestyle Enhancement Awareness Program (LEAP), 116–117

McTigue, Garrett, and Popkin, 24
Mediterranean-style diet, 105–106
Metropolitan Life Insurance Company, 45, 115
Michigan Department of Community Health, 14–16
Mitchell, Tedd, 4. *See also USA Weekend*
Mokdad, Serdula, Dietz, Bowman, Marks, and Koplan, 26–27

National Cancer Institute's 5 A Day Program, 122–123. *See also* Federal programs
National Center for Chronic Disease Prevention and Health Promotion, 27, 66
National Center for Health Statistics, 25
National Council of Negro Women, 78. *See also* Herman, Alexis
National Health and Nutrition Examination Survey (NHANES), 25, 30, 46
National Health Interview Survey, 25
National Heart, Lung, and Blood Institute, 24
National Institute of Diabetes and Digestive and Kidney Disease, 5
National Institutes of Health, 5

National Longitudinal Survey of Youth, 30
National Medical Association, 13
Native Hawaiian, 25
New Black Cultural Diet, 125, 129–150

Obesity, 24, 46. *See also* Overweight
Office of Research on Women's Health, NIH, 29, 134
Overweight, 23, 66. *See also* Obesity
Overweight and obesity in America, 25
Overweight and obesity in children, 28

Pacific Islander, 25
Peeke, Pamela, 29
Physical activity, 82
Physical fitness, 82
Physical fitness and African Americans, 86
Project Joy, 114–116

Regenstrief Health Center, 7
Robert Wood Johnson Foundation, 28

Satcher, David, 4, 24, 86
Sisters Together, 120–122. *See also* Federal programs
Slim Down Sister, 84–85, 124
Sociocultural issues, 41
Soul food, 61, 71, 142, 149. *See also* Whitehead, Tony
Soul food cookbooks, 73–78
Stack, 111
Surface structural cultural components, 138–140

Tae-Bo, 148
Thompson and Story, 32
Tutt, Brenda, 3
Tutt, Godwin, 3
Tutt, Jennifer, 4. *See also USA Weekend*

United States Department of Health and Human Services, 24, 81
Urban African Americans, 56–57, 81–82
USA Weekend, 3
USDA's Office of Experiment Stations, 68–69

Veal, Yvonnecris Smith, 13

Wagner and Howard, 47–48
Wellness Within Reach (WWR), 117–118
White, Joyce, 73–74
Whitehead, Tony, 71–72. *See also* Soul food
William Clinton Foundation, 29. *See also* Clinton, Bill
Wishard Memorial Hospital, 8
Woods, Sylvia, 73–76

About the Author

ERIC J. BAILEY is a Medical Anthropologist and Associate Professor of Anthropology and Family Medicine at East Carolina University. In earlier roles, he served as Program Director for the Masters in Public Health Program in Urban Public Health at Charles R. Drew University of Medicine and Science, as well as Health Scientist for the National Institutes of Health, National Center on Minority Health and Health Disparities.

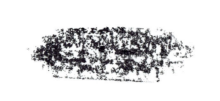